KU-245-156

PATHOLOGY OF PERIPHERAL NERVES

PATHOLOGY OF PERIPHERAL NERVES

Roy O. Weller
BSc, PhD(Lond), MD, MRCPath

Reader in Neuropathology, Faculty of Medicine,
University of Southampton

Consultant Neuropathologist to the
Wessex Regional Neurological Centre

Jorge Cervós-Navarro
MD

Professor of Neuropathology,
Director: Institut für Neuropathologie,
Klinikum Steglitz der Freien Universität, Berlin

THE BRITISH SCHOOL OF OSTEOPATHY
1-4 SUFFOLK STREET, LONDON SW1Y 4HG
TEL: 01-930 9254-8

BUTTERWORTHS
LONDON–BOSTON
Sydney–Wellington–Durban–Toronto

LROM J

THE BUTTERWORTH GROUP

United Kingdom   Butterworth & Co (Publishers) Ltd
London: 88 Kingsway, WC2B 6AB

Australia   Butterworths Pty Ltd
Sydney: 586 Pacific Highway, Chatswood NSW 2067
Also at Melbourne, Brisbane, Adelaide and Perth

Canada   Butterworth & Co (Canada) Ltd
Toronto: 2265 Midland Avenue,
Scarborough, Ontario, M1P 4S1

New Zealand   Butterworths of New Zealand Ltd
Wellington: T & W Young Building,
77–85 Customhouse Quay, 1, CPO Box 472

South Africa   Butterworth & Co (South Africa) (Pty) Ltd
Durban: 152–154 Gale Street

USA   Butterworth (Publishers) Inc
Boston: 19 Cummings Park, Woburn, Mass. 01801

All rights reserved. No part of this publication may be reproduced or transmitted in any form or by any means, including photocopying and recording, without the written permission of the copyright holder, application for which should be addressed to the Publishers. Such written permission must also be obtained before any part of this publication is stored in a retrieval system of any nature.

This book is sold subject to the Standard Conditions of Sale of Net Books and may not be resold in the UK below the net price given by the Publishers in their current price list.

First published 1977
Reprinted 1978

ISBN 0 407 00073 9

© Butterworth & Co (Publishers) Ltd 1977

Library of Congress Cataloging in Publication Data

Weller, Roy O.
Pathology of peripheral nerves.

Includes bibliographical references and index.
1. Nerves, Peripheral-Diseases.
2. Histology, Pathological I. Cervós-Navarro, J., joint author. II. Title.

RC409. W44   616.8′7   76-9758
ISBN 0-407-00073-9

Printed in England by
The Whitefriars Press Ltd,
London and Tonbridge

Preface

The purpose of writing this book is to present a synopsis of established ideas and recent progress in peripheral nerve pathology. We have also attempted to make the book into a practical manual for pathologists, neurobiologists and neurologists who wish to examine biopsy or autopsy specimens of nerve from patients or experimental animals.

Chapter 1 is a brief historical outline of the development of ideas about the structure, function and pathology of peripheral nerves. Many of the names of workers mentioned in this chapter have survived as eponymous terms. The second chapter is concerned with techniques of nerve biopsy and histological preparation; we have attempted to fit the methodology to the tissue available and to the information required. In addition to the basic methods of tissue preparation and staining, there is a section illustrating the common histological artefacts seen in peripheral nerves. Chapter 3 deals with the anatomical, histological, ultrastructural and physiological aspects of normal peripheral nerves. This is followed by an account, in Chapter 4, of the general pathological reactions of peripheral nerves. It is upon an analysis of general pathological features that many of the pathological diagnoses are made. The difficult field of clinico-pathological correlation in peripheral neuropathies is approached, in Chapter 5, mainly from the pathologist's point of view. However, an attempt is made to equate the histological and ultrastructural changes seen in specific peripheral nerve diseases with the symptomatology and electrophysiological changes. The final chapter is devoted to the histology and ultrastructure of peripheral nerve tumours and their histogenesis. The electron microscope has played a significant role in clarifying the nosology of peripheral nerve tumours, and this is one of the points that is stressed in Chapter 6.

An Appendix provides a brief guide to the examination of peripheral nerve biopsies and a summary of the main pathological features in the major peripheral nerve diseases.

The authors wish to acknowledge the material supplied by Dr G. Allt and Dr Rosalind King, and the advice and criticism from Mrs Olga Bayliss-High, Dr J. F. Hallpike, Dr P. Isaacson and Dr M. Sedgewick. Our thanks are also due to the staff of the Neuropathology Laboratory and Electron Microscope Laboratory at Southampton General Hospital. We are further indebted to the staff of the Teaching Media Centre, Southampton University, for the line drawings.

PREFACE

For that part of the book prepared in the Berlin Institute of Neuropathology the authors wish to thank Mrs C. -M. Lazaro, Mrs R. Iglesias and Mrs N. van Dooren for their fine technical work, and Dr R. Ferszt for his advice and critical comments in drafting the text.

Our special gratitude is due to Mrs Olive Huber, who typed the manuscript.

R.O.W.
J.C.-N.

Contents

1

Historical Review

Elucidation of the structure, function and pathology of peripheral nerves has proceeded in a series of steps, usually associated with advances in histological and physiological techniques. Many of the workers who made these discoveries have given their names to different structures in the peripheral nerve. Although eponymous terms are decreasing in number, many are still retained and they do appear extensively in the older literature. It seems appropriate, therefore, to give a brief account of the development of ideas about the peripheral nerve.

The gross appearance of nerve trunks was well recognized by early anatomists but a whole new field of study was opened up by the introduction of the microscope. Leeuwenhoek (1632–1723) is credited with the first description of single myelinated nerve fibres (Ranvier, 1878). In his Opera II he described nerve tubes full of liquid. The more detailed structural studies of peripheral nerves did not bear fruit, however, until the 1830s. At this time Johannes Müller had three memorable figures among his pupils in Berlin: Jacob Henle, Theodore Schwann and Robert Remak. The last two were intimately connected with the original descriptions of cellular components of peripheral nerves. Conditions of study were, apparently, far from ideal, as there were few microscopes available; Remak describes how he would pray for sunshine during the short winter days in Berlin as microscopy was not possible on dull, cloudy days (Kisch, 1954). In 1838 Remak published his thesis entitled 'Observationes anatomicae et microscopicae de systematis nervosi structura' in which he described non-myelinated nerve fibres (fibriae organicae) and the cells (Remak cells) closely associated with them. During his dissections he noticed that the myelinated fibres (tubuli primitivi) each contained 'fibra primitiva'; this structure was subsequently renamed the axis cylinder by Purkinje in 1839 (Causey, 1960). Remak's other important observation was that non-myelinated fibres arose from ganglion cells. He also noticed that cephalopods, including squids, have huge non-myelinated axons (1 mm diameter); these axons have subsequently been used in experiments on the physiology of nerve conduction (Hodgkin, 1958).

The year after Remak's thesis, Schwann (1839) published a treatise on the microscopical structure of plant and animal cells. In this work he describes how '... each nerve fibre is, throughout its entire course, a secondary cell, developed by the coalescence of primary nucleated cells'. (Translated by Henry Smith, 1847.) Schwann considered that the long chains of nucleated cells, now called Schwann cells, coalesced to form a syncytium with the formation of a continuous band of protoplasm down the centre. This polygenist concept whereby the axon was formed by the fusion of a series of separate short lengths was not shared by Remak, but it still received support until the publication of Cajal's classical studies in 1913. Schwann also observed that the nuclei of his primary cells were abundant in young developing nerve fibres but were only occasionally seen along the lengths of fully developed myelinated fibres.

In parallel with the investigation of normal nerve fibres, the effects of nerve injury were also being studied. Although Burdach (1837) observed no alteration in peripheral nerve structure 1 week after ligation, Steinbruck (1838) recorded that the nerve became more slender and atrophic. Loss of irritability and fragmentation of fibres following nerve section were recorded by Guenther and Schoen (1840). Similarly, fragmentation of the degenerating nerve fibres was observed by Nasse (1839). It was with this background of early work in Germany that Augustus Waller (1850), working in London, followed the sequence of axonal (Wallerian) degeneration in the severed glossopharyngeal and hypoglossal nerves of the frog. Having found that cutting the nerves of both sides results in the animal's death, he cut only one side and was able to observe decreased power and sensation on the affected side of the tongue. During the subsequent 12–15 days he observed the breakdown of the medullary (myelin) sheath; he described not only the granular appearance under the microscope but also the change in response of the nerve fibre components to distilled water, alkalis and ether. Two years later Waller (1852) made some further fundamental discoveries. He observed the regeneration of glossopharyngeal nerve fibres into the tongue 3–4 months after section. Furthermore, he showed that when a spinal sensory nerve is cut below the ganglion, the degeneration is not carried back to the ganglion. If, however, the ganglion itself is extirpated, the nerve degenerates. These observations supported Remak's thesis that axonal processes arose from neurones.

Although Waller (1852) considered that the nerve elements disappeared totally after degeneration, Remak (1862) observed that very thin regenerating nerves grow into old Schwann tubes which still contained degenerating myelin debris. Much of the early work on peripheral nerve was performed on unstained specimens but, about 1870, Max Schultze introduced osmic acid into histology. A 1 per cent solution of osmium tetroxide (osmic acid) is colourless but it reacts with myelin to form a black osmium compound. Using this technique to stain sections of nerve and individual teased fibres, Ranvier (1878) was able to study peripheral nerves in greater detail. Much of the two volumes of his book *Leçons sur l'histologie du Système Nerveux* is devoted to the structure of peripheral nerves. Probably Ranvier's most noteworthy contribution was his description of regular constrictions or discontinuities in the myelin sheath along the length of the fibre (*Figure 1*). Thus, he showed how the myelin is divided into segments, whereas the axon is continuous. The constrictions or 'étranglements annulaires' are now known as nodes of Ranvier and represent the short gap between segments of the myelin sheath formed by

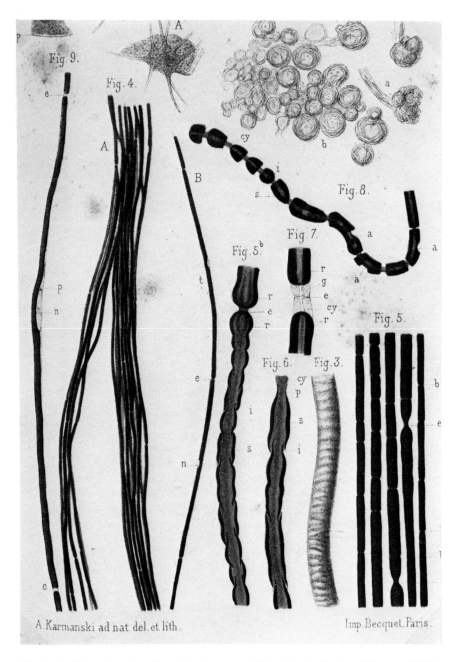

Fig. 1. An illustration from Ranvier's Leçons sur l'histologie du Système Nerveux *(1878), showing 'nodes of Ranvier' (e)*

3

consecutive Schwann cells. Ranvier also noted that the distance between each node (internodal length) was proportional to the diameter of the myelinated fibre. He suggested that the myelin might protect the axon or that it might act as an insulator in a similar way to the insulating cover on a submarine cable. The function of the nodes was discussed and he proposed that the nodal constriction might stop the semi-liquid myelin from flowing along the nerve to its lower end, or that the breaks in the sheath might allow diffusion of nutrients into the axon.

About the same time, Schmidt (1874) and Lantermann (1877) described funnel-shaped discontinuities in the internodal myelin sheath. These Schmidt–Lantermann incisures have been the source of much argument and it is only with recent electron microscope and *in vivo* light microscope studies (Hall and Williams, 1970) that they have become established entities. One of the problems has been that the incisures vary in their appearance and are sensitive to osmotic changes; often they have been dismissed as post-mortem artefact.

A significant step forward in the study of peripheral nerve pathology also occurred with the introduction of osmium staining of teased nerve fibres. Gombault (1880) described the phenomenon as 'névrite segmentaire péri-axile' (segmental demyelination) in the nerves of guinea-pigs after 8 months of lead intoxication (l'intoxication saturnine). The nerves were treated with 1 per cent osmium tetroxide to demonstrate the myelin and then with picrocarmine to stain the axons. Although the continuity of the axon was maintained, varying lengths of myelin sheath were destroyed. Similar segmental demyelination was seen following trauma. Gombault also observed thinly myelinated segments of nerve and short internodes. Soon after Gombault's original description, Meyer (1881) described the widespread segmental demyelination in patients dying with diphtheritic neuropathy. Teasing of osmium-fixed nerves still remains the most popular method for demonstrating segmental demyelination (Dyck and Gomez, 1968; Lascelles and Thomas, 1966) and diphtheria intoxication remains one of the most effective ways of inducing segmental demyelination in experimental animals (Webster *et al.*, 1961; McDonald, 1963; Cavanagh and Jacobs, 1964).

The next series of advances in the study of peripheral nerves followed the introduction of metallic impregnation techniques for staining axons by Camillo Golgi (1881) and Santiago Ramon y Cajal (1909). This was an important era in neuro-anatomy, for it was largely due to the work of Golgi and Cajal on the central nervous system that the neuronal theory was established (Cajal, 1909). Prior to this time many workers had proposed that the nervous system was a continuum and not composed of separate cells connected by synapses.

Using silver impregnation techniques, Cajal (1913) studied axon degeneration and regeneration in great detail. He showed that the proximal stump of the injured axon will usually degenerate back to the preceding node of Ranvier, or the one before. After a few hours the tip of the proximal axon stump swells to form an end bulb from which axons will sprout on about the second day. Meanwhile the axons and myelin of the distal stump have started to fragment and the debris lies mainly in the Schwann cells. Büngner (1891) described how the Schwann cells in the distal stump form rows along the nerve (Zellbänder, or bands of Büngner). However, Büngner belonged to the 'polygenist' school and proposed that, during regeneration, the axoplasm appeared in the centre of each Schwann cell and finally fused to form a

4

continuous axon. Cajal was able to show that each axon regenerated by growing from the proximal stump along the bands of Büngner and retained its continuity with the neuronal cell body throughout.

The induction of chromatolysis in the neurone cell body by axon section had been observed by Nissl in 1892. He evulsed the facial nerve from the stylomastoid foramen and then stained sections of the facial nucleus with cresyl violet. Some days after the axotomy the motor neurones swelled, the nuclei became eccentric and the staining intensity of the cytoplasmic 'Nissl substance' decreased.

During the last 30–40 years there has been a parallel acquisition of information about the structure and function of peripheral nerves using several techniques. Schmidt and Bear (1939) really opened this modern era with their X-ray diffraction and polarized light studies of myelin. They reached the conclusion that myelin is composed of concentric sheets of protein interspersed with layers of lipoid so as to form structures which are repeated periodically in a radial direction. This structure is basically a stack of membranes with the bimolecular lipid form proposed by Gerter and Grendell in 1926, and Davson and Danielli (1943). Subsequent electron microscope studies of fresh myelin (Fernández-Moran, 1950) have confirmed its lamellar structure. Molecular models for myelin were proposed by Finean (1953) on the basis of X-ray diffraction and electron microscope data. He arranged the polar phospholipids as bimolecular leaflets with the polar ends of the molecules associated with hydrophilic protein layer. Cholesterol was incorporated into the hydrophobic part of the structure. Variations on this model have been put forward by Vanderheuvel (1965).

As with most other tissues, electron microscope studies have added an immense amount of detailed information about the structure of peripheral nerves. Geren (1954) showed, in developing chick nerves, that the myelin sheath is formed from the compaction of layers of Schwann cell membrane arranged in a spiral around the axon. Fine-structural studies of permanganate-fixed material led Robertson (1961) to formulate a 'unit membrane' theory. He found that cell membranes exhibited a trilaminar structure, the outer layers of which fused during the compaction of a myelin sheath. Gradually the complex structural characteristics of the node of Ranvier and paranodal regions emerged (Elvin, 1961; Landon and Williams, 1963; Williams and Landon, 1963). Following the introduction of glutaraldehyde as a primary fixative (Sabatini, Bensch and Barrnett, 1963), the structure of the axon and its high content of microtubules and filaments could be more adequately studied.

Advances in peripheral nerve physiology occurred in various fields. Weiss and Hiscoe (1948) observed that axons became swollen proximal to the compression of the nerve by an arterial sleeve and proposed that axoplasm flowed from the cell body of the neurone to the distal end of the nerve. The introduction of radioactive isotope techniques and histochemically or ultrastructurally identifiable markers (Barondes, 1967) has led to a better understanding of the rates of axoplasmic transport and the mechanisms involved (Ochs, 1972; Kristensson and Olsson, 1973).

There have also been major advances in the electrophysiological investigation of isolated nerve fibres and of intact nerve trunks in the last 30 years. Young (1936) rediscovered the very large non-myelinated nerve fibres in cephalopods. The giant axon of the squid can be emptied of cytoplasm so that

5

both the inside and the outside of the limiting membrane can be studied. In this way, the mechanisms involved in membrane depolarization and impulse propagation could be investigated (Hodgkin, 1958). The basic differences between the continuous passage of an impulse along the non-myelinated nerve and the saltatory conduction of myelinated fibres was emphasized by Huxley and Stämpfli (1949) in their studies on isolated frog sciatic nerve.

The introduction of techniques for measuring nerve conduction in intact animals and human patients was a major advance in the study of normal physiology and peripheral nerve diseases. In the 1930s electromyography involved the recording of electrical activity in resting and active muscles (Gilliatt, 1966). Hodes, Larrabee and German (1948), however, introduced techniques for measuring nerve conduction. They measured conduction velocities in motor nerves by stimulating various peripheral nerves and recording the response with electrodes placed over the relevant muscles. Subsequently Dawson and Scott (1949) measured conduction velocities in sensory nerves with electrodes placed on the skin. It was soon found that conduction velocities were reduced in regenerating nerves following injury (Hodes *et al.*, 1948), in polyneuropathies (Henriksen, 1956) and in nerve compression (Simpson, 1956); the most dramatic slowing, however, is associated with segmental demyelination (McDonald, 1963). These findings added impetus to the renewed interest in the study of teased fibres, where the relationship between internodal lengths and fibre diameters was established in developing and regenerating nerve fibres (Vizoso and Young, 1948; Thomas and Young, 1949; Lascelles and Thomas, 1966). Many neuropathies are now studied by combined clinical electrophysiology and peripheral nerve biopsy. Techniques have been developed also for the measurement of conduction velocities and compound action potentials in isolated lengths of nerve biopsy which are subsequently studied histologically (Dyck, Lambert and Nichols, 1971).

Sophistication of biochemical and histochemical techniques for lipids and proteins (Adams, 1965; Davison and Peters, 1970) during the last few decades has led to a more complete understanding of the metabolism of normal and diseased peripheral nerves. Similarly, the advances in the pharmacology of neurotransmitters and the physiology of neuromuscular transmission are too many to enumerate individually. These fields have benefited greatly from the introduction of intracellular electrode and iontophoretic techniques whereby minute quantities of pharmacologically active agents or radioactive material can be administered at physiologically active sites (Globus, Lux and Schubert, 1968).

No attempt has been made in this chapter to give an exhaustive history of the development of ideas about the nerve fibre. Opinions differ about what is important in the growth of knowledge, just as many of the discoveries recounted here took many years to gain acceptance. The historical background to various structures, functions and disease processes discussed in the rest of the book will not be emphasized, as more prominence will be given to modern concepts and recent developments.

REFERENCES

Adams, C. W. M. (1965). *Neurohistochemistry*. Amsterdam; Elsevier.

Barondes, S. H. (1967). 'Axoplasmic transport'. *Neurosciences Research Program Bulletin*, **5**, 307.

Büngner, O. von (1891). 'Ueber die Degeneration und Regenerations-vorgänge am Nerven nach Verletzungen.' *Arb. Path. Inst. Marburg*, **3**, 165.

Burdach, E. (1837). In *Beitrag zur Mikroskopischer Anatomie der Nerven*. Königsberg.

Cajal, S. R. y. (1909). *Histologie du système nerveux de l'homme et des vertébrés*. Paris; A. Maloine.

Cajal, S. R. y (1913). *Degeneration and Regeneration of the Nervous System*. English translation 1928. London; Oxford University Press.

Causey, G. (1960). In *The Cell of Schwann*. Edinburgh and London; Livingstone.

Cavanagh, J. B. and Jacobs, J. M. (1964). 'Some quantitative aspects of diphtheritic neuropathy'. *Br. J. Exp. Pathol.*, **45**, 309.

Davison, A. N. and Peters, A. (1970). In *Myelination*. Springfield, Illinois; Charles C. Thomas.

Davson, H. and Danielli, J. F. (1943). In *The Permeability of Natural Membranes*. Cambridge.

Dawson, D. G. and Scott, J. W. (1949). 'The recording of nerve action potentials through the skin in man'. *J. Neurol. Neurosurg. Psychiat.*, **12**, 259.

Dyck, P. J. and Gomez, M. R. (1968). 'Segmental demyelination in Dejerine–Sottas disease'. *Mayo Clin. Proc.*, **43**, 280.

Dyck, P. J., Lambert, E. H. and Nichols, P. C. (1971). 'Quantitative measurement of sensation related to compound action potential and number and sizes of myelinated and unmyelinated fibres of sural nerve in health, Friedreich's ataxia, hereditary sensory neuropathy and tabes dorsalis'. In *Handbook of Electroencephalography and Clinical Neurophysiology*, Vol. 9, p. 83. Amsterdam; Elsevier.

Elfvin, L.-G. (1961). 'The ultrastructure of the nodes of Ranvier in cat sympathetic nerve fibres'. *J. Ultrastruct. Res.*, **5**, 374.

Fernández-Morán, H. (1950). 'Electron microscope observations on the structure of the myelinated nerve fibre sheath.' *Exp. Cell Res.*, **1**, 143.

Finean, J. B. (1953). 'Phospholipid–cholesterol complex in the structure of myelin'. *Experimentia*, **9**, 17.

Geren, B. B. (1954). 'The formation from the Schwann cell surface of myelin in the peripheral nerves of chick embryos'. *Exp. Cell Res.*, **7**, 558.

Gilliatt, R. W. (1966). 'Disorders of peripheral nerve'. *J. Roy. Coll. Phcns. London*, **1**, 50.

Globus, A., Lux, H. D. and Schubert, P. (1968). 'Somadendritic spread of intracellularly injected tritiated glycine in cat spinal motor neurones'. *Brain Res.*, **11**, 440.

Golgi, C. (1881). 'Sulla struttura delle fibre nervose midollate periferiche e central'. *Arch. Sci. Med.*, **4**, 221.

Gombault, A. (1880). 'Contribution à l'étude anatomique de la névrite parenchymateuse subaiguë et chronique—Névrite segmentaire péri-axile.' *Arch. Neurol. (Paris)*, **1**, 11.

Guenther and Schoen (1840). 'Versuche und Bemerkungen über Regeneration der Nerven und Abhängigkeit der peripherischen Nerven von der Centralorganen.' *Müller Arch.*, 270.

Hall, S. M. and Williams, P. L. (1970). 'Studies on the "incisures" of Schmidt and Lanterman'. *J. Cell Sci.*, **6**, 767.

Henriksen, J. D. (1956). 'Conduction velocity of motor nerves in normal subjects and patients with neuromuscular disorders'. M.S. Thesis, University of Minnesota (quoted by Gilliatt, 1966).

Hodes, R., Larrabee, M. C. and German, W. J. (1948). 'The human electromyogram in response to nerve stimulation and the conduction velocity of motor axons; studies on normal and on injured peripheral nerves'. *Arch. Neurol. Psychiat.*, **60**, 340.

Hodgkin, A. L. (1958). 'Ionic movements and electrical activity in giant nerve fibres'. *Proc. Roy. Soc. B*, **148**, 1.

Huxley, A. F. and Stämpfli, R. (1949). 'Evidence of saltatory conduction in peripheral myelinated nerve fibres'. *J. Physiol.*, **108**, 315.

Kisch, B. Z. (1954). 'Forgotten leaders in medicine'. *Trans. Am. Phil. Soc.*, **44**, 227.

Kristensson, K. and Olsson, Y. (1973). 'Diffusion pathways and retrograde axonal transport of protein tracers in peripheral nerves'. *Progr. Neurobiol.*, **1**, 85.

Landon, D. N. and Williams, P. L. (1963). 'Ultrastructure of the node of Ranvier'. *Nature (London)*, **199**, 575.

REFERENCES

Lanterman, A. J. (1877). 'Ueber den feineren Bander markhaltigen Nervenfasern'. *Arch. Mikrosk. Anat.*, **13**, 1.

Lascelles, R. G. and Thomas, P. K. (1966). 'Changes due to age in internodal length in the sural nerve in man'. *J. Neurol. Neurosurg. Psychiat.*, **29**, 40.

McDonald, W. I. (1963). 'The effects of experimental demyelination on conduction in peripheral nerve: a histological and electrophysiological study. II. Electrophysiological observations'. *Brain*, **86**, 501.

Meyer, P. (1881). 'Anatomische Untersuchungen über diphtheritische Lähmung'. *Virchows Arch. Pathol. Anat.*, **85**, 181.

Nasse (1839). 'Ueber die Veränderungen der Nervenfasern nach ihrer Durchschneidung'. *Müller Arch.*, 405.

Nissl, F. (1892). Über die Veränderungen der Ganglienzellen am Facialiskern des Kaninchens nach Ausreissung der Nerven'. *Allgem. Z. Psychiatr.*, **48**, 197.

Ochs, S. (1972). 'Fast transport of materials in mammalian nerve fibres'. *Science, N.Y.*, **176**, 252.

Ranvier, L. (1878). In *Leçons sur l'histologie du système nerveux*. Paris; F. Savy.

Remak, R. (1838). In *Observationes anatomicae et microscopicae de systematis nervosi structura*. Berlin.

Remak, R. (1862). 'Ueber die Wiedererzeugung von Nervenfasern'. *Virchows Arch.*, **23**, 441.

Robertson, J. D. (1961). 'The unit membrane'. In *Electron Microscopy in Anatomy*. London; Edward Arnold.

Sabatini, D. D., Bensch, K. and Barrnett, R. J. (1963). 'Cytochemistry and electron microscopy. The preservation of cellular ultrastructure and enzymatic activity by aldehyde fixation'. *J. Cell Biol.*, **17**, 19.

Schmidt, F. O. and Bear, R. S. (1939). 'The ultrastructure of the nerve axon sheath'. *Biol. Rev.*, **14**, 27.

Schmidt, H. D. (1874). 'On the construction of the dark or double-bordered nerve fibre'. *Monthly Microscopy J. (London)*, **11**, 200.

Schwann, Th. von (1839). *Mikroskopische Untersuchungen über die Uebereinstimmung in der Structur und dem Wachsthum der Thiere und Pflanzen*. Berlin; G. E. Reimer.

Schwann, Th. von (1847). *Microscopical Researches into the Accordance in the Structure and Growth of Animals and Plants*. Translated by Henry Smith. London; Sydenham Society.

Simpson, J. A. (1956). 'Electrical signs in the diagnosis of carpal tunnel and related syndromes'. *J. Neurol. Neurosurg. Psychiat.*, **19**, 275.

Steinbruck (1838). In *De Nervorum Regeneratione*. Berlin.

Thomas, P. K. and Young, J. Z. (1949). 'Internode lengths in the nerves of fishes'. *J. Anat. (London)*, **83**, 336.

Vanderheuvel, F. A. (1965). 'Structural studies of biological membranes'. *Ann. N.Y. Acad. Sci.*, **122**, Part 1, 57.

Vizoso, A. D. and Young, J. Z. (1948). 'Internode length and fibre diameter in developing and regenerating nerves'. *J. Anat.*, **82**, 110.

Waller, A. (1850). 'Experiments on the section of the glossopharyngeal and hypoglossal nerves of the frog and observations of the alterations produced thereby in the structure of their primitive fibres'. *Phil. Trans. Roy. Soc.*, **140**, 423.

Waller, A. (1852). 'Sur la reproduction des nerfs et sur la structure et les fonctions des ganglions spinaux'. *Arch. Anat. Physiol. Wissenschaft. Med. (Müller's Arch.)* 392.

Webster, H. de F., Spiro, D., Waksman, B. and Adams, R. (1961). 'Phase and electron microscopic studies of experimental demyelination. II. Schwann cell changes in guinea-pig sciatic nerves during experimental diphtheritic neuritis'. *J. Neuropath. Exp. Neurol.*, **20**, 5.

Weiss, P. and Hiscoe, H. B. (1948). 'Experiments on mechanisms of nerve growth'. *J. Exp. Zool.*, **107**, 315.

Williams, P. L. and Landon, D. N. (1963). 'Paranodal apparatus of peripheral myelinated nerve fibres of mammals'. *Nature (London)*, **198**, 670.

Young, J. Z. (1936). 'The giant nerve fibres and epistellar body of cephalopods'. *Quart. J. Microscop. Sci.*, **78**, 367.

2

Techniques of Peripheral Nerve Biopsy and Histological Preparation

INTRODUCTION

There are three main sources of peripheral nerve tissue usually available to the pathologist: elective biopsies from patients, peripheral nerve material obtained at autopsy and specimens from experimental animals. All sources have their advantages but should be approached differently if the maximum amount of information is to be obtained from the tissue. Patients with peripheral neuropathies should be thoroughly investigated clinically before a biopsy is done so that any special techniques or fixatives that are required can be prepared. Great care must be taken with the biopsy technique, as the nerve can be easily damaged by rough handling either by the surgeon or by the pathologist. The introduction of artefact in this way has been responsible in the past for several misleading reports of histological changes in peripheral neuropathies. If possible, part of each nerve biopsy should be embedded in epoxy resin for the preparation of 1 μm sections and electron microscopy. Other parts of the biopsy can be preserved for teasing and paraffin embedding. Biopsy material is ideal for enzyme and lipid studies, by both biochemical and histochemical techniques. Although the amount of tissue available at autopsy is usually very much greater than that obtained at biopsy, the methods suitable for studying autopsy tissue are limited. What this means in practical terms is that fine structural details of peripheral nerves and labile biochemical processes must be studied in biopsy material, whereas the distribution throughout the body of histologically recognizable peripheral nerve damage can be documented in autopsy material. For example, the cytological identification of the cells forming the 'onion-bulb' whorls in hypertrophic neuropathy was only possible by the electron microscopical study of biopsy material. The distribution of vascular lesions in peripheral nerves, however, is only possible when long lengths of nerve are examined at autopsy (Dyck, Conn and Okazaki, 1972).

Some neuropathies only affect motor nerves or nerve roots; it is therefore not possible to study the changes extensively in biopsy specimens. A few successful post-mortem studies have been carried out at electron microscope level, but usually the tissue preservation is far from ideal and the findings may be misleading.

Study of the basic pathological processes in peripheral nerves is done most satisfactorily in experimental animals. The time intervals between the pathological insult and the study of the results can be strictly regulated. Ideal fixation may be attained by whole body perfusion with either buffered formalin or Susa fixative for light microscopy, or with glutaraldehyde for electron microscopy. If material is required for biochemical estimations, it can be obtained in a very fresh state. By correlating the information obtained from human biopsy and autopsy material with findings in experimental animals, a more complete picture of the pathology of peripheral neuropathies has emerged.

TECHNIQUES OF PERIPHERAL NERVE BIOPSY

Choice of nerve

The most suitable nerves for biopsy are those which are moderately involved in the neuropathy; nerves that are severely involved may be too damaged to reveal useful information about the original disease process. Ideally, the nerve should be either purely motor or purely sensory; it should be constant in its anatomical site and easily accessible so that, if necessary, a 4–5 cm length of nerve may be obtained. Some nerves are often damaged by entrapment—for example, the ulnar, median and lateral popliteal nerves—and they should be avoided if the purpose of the biopsy is to study a polyneuropathy. Electrophysiological studies should be carried out before the biopsy, and it is very useful to have physiological and histological data on the same nerve.

Impairment of neurological function in peripheral neuropathies is usually more pronounced in the distal nerves in the lower extremities. For this reason together with those mentioned above, the sural (sensory) and the deep peroneal (motor) nerves are often chosen for biopsy. The sural nerve is more commonly used, as its removal causes only minor sensory loss and paraesthesiae over the lateral side of the foot; these symptoms usually disappear after a few months (Dyck and Lofgren, 1966). Biopsies of motor nerves may be difficult to justify, as the patient may be left with a permanent weakness of the denervated muscle. A more practical solution is to biopsy a muscle in its motor end-plate region and to examine the intramuscular nerves. An estimate of the extent of denervation can also be obtained from the muscle biopsy. Other nerves are accessible to biopsy; for example, the occipital nerve and the lateral cutaneous nerve of the forearm. One of the disadvantages of biopsies from these less usual sites is that control data are not as readily available. The sural nerve, on the other hand, is well documented both in normal individuals at varying ages

(Lascelles and Thomas, 1966; Dyck *et al.*, 1968; Ochoa and Mair, 1969) and in a variety of pathological conditions.

Technique of nerve biopsy

Unfixed peripheral nerves are very susceptible to damage produced by crushing during excision; myelin sheaths are particularly vulnerable, as they are almost liquid in consistency in the unfixed state. Extreme care must, therefore, be taken by the surgeon during the removal of the nerve if artefact is to be avoided. For this reason peripheral nerve biopsies should be performed by an experienced surgeon after full consultation with the pathologist and preferably in his presence.

The sural nerve contains sensory fibres which supply the skin of the lateral side of the foot and heel; it passes behind and below the lateral malleolus, where it breaks up into several cutaneous branches. The patient lies prone on the operating table with the ankle supported and slightly everted. A 5–6 cm incision is made under local anaesthesia in the furrow just in front of the tendo achilles ending just above and behind the lateral malleolus. Bleeding points should be tied and no diathermy should be used. By careful sharp dissection the lesser saphenous vein is exposed deep to the deep fascia. The sural nerve at this point is a bundle of fascicles tightly bound together in an elliptical white nerve trunk 2–3 mm in diameter. It is usually behind and deep to the lesser saphenous vein and bound to the vein by loose connective tissue. Branches of the vein crossing the nerve should be divided and the connective tissue between the vein and the nerve carefully incised. As little adipose tissue as possible should be left attached to the nerve, but vigorous cleaning or even touching the nerve should be avoided completely. It is important that haemostasis should be rigorously maintained by clipping and tying even small vessels, as dabbing the nerve with a swab produces crush artefact. The whole width of the nerve trunk may be taken as a biopsy or just part of the nerve. In this latter technique of fascicular biopsy (Dyck and Lofgren, 1966) only part of the width of the nerve is cut across and this is gently separated by sharp dissection from the main trunk of the nerve. Fascicular nerve biopsy reduces the degree of neurological deficit and is suitable for most purposes, but it may not be possible to examine the epineurial arteries adequately by this technique.

For most purposes of histological investigation a 3–4 cm length of nerve is sufficient. If conduction studies are performed on isolated nerve segments, however, 5–8 cm is required (Dyck and Lofgren, 1966).

Directly the nerve has been excised, it should be handed with the forceps directly to the histologist and placed on dental wax. If the nerve is placed on gauze, it will stick firmly and damage will occur as it is picked free. It is useful at this time to note whether the nerve is a normal white colour or whether it is thin and grey with the tough texture of long-standing axonal degeneration. The thickened nerves from a patient with hypertrophic neuropathy may have a distinctive grey and gelatinous appearance. The nerve is gently stretched on a piece of dry card so that the minute transverse ridges in the epineurium disappear; then the very ends of the nerve are pressed on to the card so that they adhere. In this way the nerve is kept straight during fixation and it is easier to prepare and to examine histologically. Alternatively, the nerve can be stretched by suspending it in a bottle of fixative with a 2 g weight attached to its lower end (Dyck and Lofgren, 1966).

Glutaraldehyde is probably the best all-purpose primary fixative for electron microscopy. Tissue for light microscopy is best fixed in buffered formal saline for general histological purposes; some histochemical techniques require unfixed tissue.

Autopsy material

The use of autopsy material for the study of peripheral neuropathies presents the investigator with a far greater choice of material. Whole nerves can be examined from roots to distal termination, and this is particularly valuable in any search for isolated vascular or inflammatory lesions. Care should still be exercised in the removal of the nerve, as crushing will cause artefact. Short lengths of nerve should be slightly stretched and placed on card so that the specimen remains straight. If the nerve is thick, a central window may be cut in the card and the nerve suspended across it to allow better access of the fixative. Epoxy resin preparations of autopsy material for light and electron microscopy are usually not very satisfactory, as the resolution attained by these techniques emphasizes even the slightest post-mortem autolysis. The ultrastructural study of viruses, e.g. herpes zoster, or some lipid inclusions is still possible in autopsy material. Much useful information may be obtained from paraffin sections of autopsy material and from teased preparations. Histochemical methods for lipids and proteins are usually applicable to post-mortem nerves, but many of the enzyme techniques may be unreliable (Adams, 1965).

Tissue from experimental animals

As with human autopsy material, tissue from many sites may be studied. Optimal histological preservation may be attained by perfusion of fixative through the heart of an anaesthetized animal. It is important to avoid intravascular clotting during perfusions, especially when the tissue is to be used for electron microscopy. Various precautions can be taken. Heparin can be injected either intramuscularly or intravenously 10–15 min before the perfusion begins. Better perfusions are usually attained if the fluid is introduced at systolic pressure through the left ventricle at a flow rate similar to that of the blood or a little higher. A good outlet from the venous side of the heart is ensured by amputating the right auricular appendage. The blood can be washed out of the vascular system if necessary by saline or by paraformaldehyde in the case of glutaraldehyde perfusions. After a good perfusion, the animal should be rigid; specimens of nerves, dorsal roots and ganglia are more easily removed well fixed and undamaged from a perfused animal. Biopsies of limb nerves and other superficial nerves, however, may also be taken from anaesthetized animals.

TABLE 1
Investigation of Peripheral Nerve Tissue

	Epoxy resin sections	Paraffin sections	Teased preparations	Histochemical techniques	Biochemical preparations
Fixation or preservation	(a) Glutaraldehyde or paraformaldehyde (b) Post-fix in OsO$_4$	(a) Formalin (b) Susa	(a) Glutaraldehyde or formalin (b) Post-fix in OsO$_4$	(a) Unfixed or (b) Brief fixation in formalin, paraformaldehyde or glutaraldehyde (for EM)	Unfixed fresh tissue frozen, or quenched in liquid nitrogen
Type of preparation	Small nerve biopsies; TS and LS	Large specimens of nerve, biopsy and autopsy material	Individual nerve fibres	(a) Cryostat or frozen sections (b) Teased preparations	(a) Homogenates (b) Separation of components by centrifugation
Features of the nerve to be investigated	*Light microscopy* TS (and LS) (a) Quantification of myelinated (and non-myelinated) nerves (b) Axon: myelin sheath ratios (c) Cell components of nerve fascicles (d) Autoradiography *Electron microscopy* TS and LS (a) Ultrastructure of nerve components (b) Quantification of non-myelinated fibres (c) Tumours—cell identification	(a) Cell components and myelinated fibres; TS and LS (b) Connective tissue of nerve (c) Vessels (d) Inflammatory cells (e) Tumours—histological patterns	(a) Internodal lengths and fibre diameters of individual fibres (b) Detection of current or past segmental demyelination and axonal degeneration (c) Histochemical studies on Schwann cells and axons	(a) Lipids, proteins and mucosubstances in normal and degenerating nerves (b) Abnormal lipids (e.g. sulphatide in metachromatic leukodystrophy) (c) Enzymes and neurotransmitters	(a) Chemical composition of nerve components (b) Enzyme abnormalities (c) Abnormal lipid components (d) Isotope labelling of nerve constituents

NERVE BIOPSY AND HISTOLOGY

TECHNIQUES FOR THE INVESTIGATION OF PERIPHERAL NERVE TISSUE

Various techniques will reveal different aspects of peripheral nerve structure and metabolism (*Table 1*). It is, therefore, important to ensure appropriate primary fixation and handling of the tissue. In addition to applying the most suitable techniques to the nerves, it is also essential that the specimens be properly orientated during the embedding procedure in order to give either exact transverse or exact longitudinal sections. Oblique sections are difficult to interpret and often misleading.

Histological techniques for peripheral nerves

Epoxy resin embedding

This method of tissue preparation is ideal for biopsy material and for perfused animal tissue. The nerves should be fixed in 3 per cent glutaraldehyde or paraformaldehyde in either phosphate or cacodylate buffer at pH 7·4 for 4 h and then washed overnight in 0·2 M cacodylate buffer at pH 7·4 containing 7·5 per cent sucrose (Glauert, 1975). Following the primary fixation, excessive epineurial fat should be trimmed from the nerve and portions of nerve up to 1 mm thick selected for transverse or longitudinal

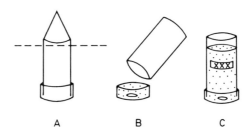

Fig. 2. *The top is cut from a Beem capsule (A); the specimen is placed in the resin-filled lid (B); lastly, the rest of the capsule is replaced and filled with resin and the label inserted (C)*

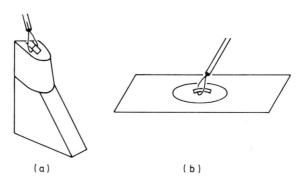

(a) (b)

Fig. 3

14

section. Often the nerve trunk can be cut into flat transverse slices 2–3 mm in diameter and 1 mm thick. The nerve is then post-fixed in osmium tetroxide (Dalton, Palade or Millonig fixative) for 2–4 h, dehydrated in alcohol and propylene oxide and embedded in Araldite. Care should be taken to embed the nerve with the correct orientation, either in a rubber mould or in the flat lid of a shaped plastics 'BEEM' capsule (*Figure 2*).

One μm sections of epoxy resin-embedded material can be cut for light microscopy with glass knives on an ultratome. Sections are floated on water in a boat attached to the knife (*Figure 3a*) and then transferred to a drop of warm water on a slide (*Figure 3b*) with a stout bristle loop. Flattening of the sections is achieved by draining the water from the slide, then adding a drop of xylene to each section and drying the slide on a hotplate at 60°C.

Staining of epoxy resin sections

Several techniques have been developed for staining 1 μm sections. Two useful methods for peripheral nerves are toluidine blue and a combined toluidine blue and carbol fuchsin stain. Araldite preparations stain consistently with less background staining than epon sections.

Method
(1) Dry sections on to slide.
(2) Remove resin with sodium methoxide (about 30 s). (This step is not necessary if only toluidine blue is used.)
(3) Wash in absolute alcohol.
(4) Wash in distilled water.
(5) Stain on hotplate at 60 °C with 1 per cent toluidine blue in 1 per cent borax. The slide should be flooded with stain and left on the hotplate until the mixture steams.
(6) Wash in water.
(7) Cover slide with distilled water and add 2–3 drops of carbol fuchsin and mix (carbol fuchsin consists of: basic fuchsin, 1 g; absolute alcohol, 10 ml; 5 per cent aqueous phenol, 100 ml). The staining time is usually a few seconds and should be monitored under the microscope.
(8) Wash with distilled water.
(9) Blot dry and mount.

Although toluidine blue alone is suitable for most histological studies and myelinated fibre measurements, the carbol fuchsin modification has the advantage that it stains the endoneurial connective tissue pink and allows better definition of cellular processes.

Difficulty may be encountered with flattening transverse sections of nerves, especially the epineurium. Some improvement may be obtained by trimming as much fat and connective tissue as possible from the block and by cutting thinner sections.

Electron microscopy

Areas for electron microscopic study can be selected from the 1 μm sections and the block trimmed accordingly. Standard uranyl acetate and lead citrate

(Hayat, 1970) staining of ultrathin sections produces the best general contrast for electron microscopy. In addition to the usefulness of electron microscopy in the identification of the cell components in peripheral nerves, it is really the only accurate way of estimating non-myelinated fibre number and size.

Paraffin embedding

Although material embedded in paraffin is not suitable for high-resolution microscopy, the tissue should still be gently handled until it is well fixed. Buffered formalin is an all-purpose fixative for paraffin embedding and Susa gives good preservation especially when used for perfusion. Tissue fixed in glutaraldehyde is brittle and difficult to cut in paraffin. Fleming's solution containing chromate and osmium tetroxide can be used as a primary fixative (Cavanagh and Jacobs, 1964) for the demonstration of myelin sheaths in paraffin sections without further staining.

As far as possible transverse or longitudinal sections should be cut. Apart from general histological stains such as haematoxylin and eosin and Van Gieson, there are several axonal stains (Glees and Marsland, Palmgren) and myelin stains (Loyez, Heidenhain's haematoxylin) that may be employed (Drury and Wallington, 1967). Luxol fast blue is often used for myelin in peripheral nerves but unfortunately it also stains the connective tissue.

Teased preparations

Osmium-fixed preparations. Teasing of nerves is the best and perhaps the only way of adequately examining lengths of individual peripheral nerve fibres for evidence of segmental demyelination and axonal degeneration. Nodal gaps at the nodes of Ranvier, internodal lengths of myelin sheath and fibre diameters can all be measured in osmium-fixed teased fibres or in formalin-fixed preparation stained with Sudan black B (Cavanagh and Jacobs, 1964). Irregularities in normal myelin sheaths and in the myelin sheaths in some peripheral neuropathies can also be detected in osmium-fixed teased fibres.

Lengths of nerve of 1–2 cm are fixed primarily in formalin (24 h) or glutaraldehyde (2–4 h) and then 1 mm diameter fascicles are post-fixed in 1 per cent osmium tetroxide (2–4 h), dehydrated in alcohol and propylene oxide as for electron microscopy and then soaked overnight in Araldite from which the accelerator has been omitted. This procedure softens the nerves and allows the fibres to be teased apart. The final separation of fibres is performed with sharp sewing needles on a glass slide in complete Araldite under a dissecting microscope. Practice is required to separate long lengths of individual nerve fibres and a less damaged preparation may be obtained if a sheath of fibres is separated only at one end like a horse's tail. When the fibres have been teased, they are covered by a cover slip and the Araldite is hardened in a 60 °C oven.

Histochemistry of teased fibres. Various enzyme and lipid histochemical methods can be applied to nerve and the reaction products detected in teased nerve fibres (Kalyanaraman and Finlayson, 1969; Morgan-Hughes and Engel, 1968; Weller and Nester, 1972). If the perineurium is incised, the nerve fibres can be gently spread out prior to application of the histochemical technique.

The stained specimens are soaked in 66 per cent glycerine prior to teasing and the teased preparations mounted either in 66 per cent glycerine or glycerine jelly.

NADH—tetrazolium reductase staining is useful for outlining Schwann cytoplasm (Morgan-Hughes and Engel, 1968; Weller and Nester, 1972). Other enzyme techniques, including cholinesterase (Kalyanaraman and Finlayson, 1969) and acid phosphatase (Weller and Nester, 1972), have been applied to normal and abnormal nerves. The myelin sheath can be visualized by polarized light (Weller and Nester, 1972). Oil red O staining combined with a haematoxylin nuclear stain (Jacobs, 1967) is also a very useful technique for studying the cytology of teased nerves.

Histochemistry of peripheral nerves

Histochemistry is particularly useful for localizing lipids, proteins, polysaccharides and sites of enzyme activity within normal and abnormal nerves. Various techniques can be applied to frozen sections or teased preparations for light microscopy, and some methods are suitable for electron microscopy. Techniques may not be specific for one particular lipid or protein, and identification of a particular substance may require several histochemical methods together with selective extraction or blocking procedures. Enzyme techniques, on the whole, are usually more specific.

A brief outline of techniques that are useful in the study of peripheral nerves is given here, but more comprehensive accounts of the methods and their chemical bases are given by Adams (1965) and Pearse (1968, 1972).

Lipid histochemistry

Normal myelin. Lipids account for over half the dry weight of myelin and consist mostly of cholesterol, phospholipids (sphingomyelin and lecithin) and cerebroside (a glycolipid). Cryostat sections of fresh tissue are preferred; they can be post-fixed in formal calcium (1 per cent calcium acetate in 10 per cent formalin) when appropriate (Adams and Bayliss, 1975). Material previously fixed in formalin can be sectioned on a freezing microtome (e.g. Pelcool). Most of the lipid is removed during processing of paraffin-embedded tissue.

Cholesterol can be localized histochemically by the perchloric acid naphthoquinone (PAN) method (Adams, 1961) and by the Schultz technique (Lewis and Lobban, 1961). Sudan black stains phospholipids and glycolipids in the normal myelin sheath as well as triglycerides in the epineurial adipose tissue and the cholesterol esters of degenerating myelin.

There are more specific methods for detecting phospholipids. Baker's acid haematin technique (Adams, 1965) stains choline-containing phospholipids (lecithin and sphingomyelin) black. The ester linkages in lecithin are hydrolysed by alkalis, whereas sphingomyelin has an amide bond which is alkali-resistant; therefore only sphingomyelin stains in tissue sections with Baker's acid haematin following NAOH hydrolysis (NAOH—Baker's acid haematin technique).

Phosphoglycerides (e.g. lecithin but not sphingomyelin) stain red or purple

17

with the gold hydroxamate technique (Gallyas, 1963; Adams, Bayliss and Ibrahim, 1963a). This technique has been adapted for electron microscopy (Weller *et al.*, 1965).

There is no specific stain for the characteristic myelin glycolipid cerebroside, but, because it contains a sugar moiety, it can be stained by a modified periodic acid Schiff (PAS) technique (Adams, Davison and Gregson, 1963b). Sections treated with chloroform—methanol (2:1 v/v) lose their cerebroside; the difference in staining between the extracted and non-extracted sections of myelin is accounted for mainly by the cerebroside content.

Degenerating myelin. Long-standing myelin loss can be detected histochemically by reduced staining of normal myelin lipids within the nerve. However, during the process of myelin breakdown and removal of the debris there are distinct changes in the myelin lipids, the most notable of which is the esterification of cholesterol to form cholesterol esters. Several staining methods for degenerating myelin rely largely on the physical properties of the cholesterol esters. Oil red O and Sudan red stain globular lipids, including cholesterol esters, bright red, whereas normal myelin is only stained lightly. Cholesterol esters are stained black by the osmium in the osmium tetroxide α-naphthylamine (OTAN) technique (Adams, 1965) and in the Marchi technique. In both these methods the osmiophilia of normal myelin is blocked by potassium chlorate or chromate.

Triglycerides also stain black with the OTAN and Marchi techniques. Although in practice there is little triglyceride in the degenerating nerve except in the epineurium, there is a specific lipase technique for triglyceride (Adams *et al.*, 1966) which would distinguish them from cholesterol esters. The PAN method for cholesterol also stains cholesterol esters.

Abnormal lipids accumulate within the nervous system in the sphingolipidoses. In the gangliosidoses the lipids are mainly demonstrable in the neuronal cell bodies of the brain and in the peripheral ganglia, e.g. in the gut wall (Bodian and Lake, 1963). Diagnosis may therefore be made by identifying the abnormal lipids in the central nervous system, appendix or rectal biopsy. Enzyme defects may be detected in cultured fibroblasts from the skin of patients with lipid storage diseases (Bearn, 1972).

Metachromatic leukodystrophy (sulphatide lipidosis) is the main lipidosis where abnormal amounts of lipid accumulate in the peripheral nerves. The sulphatide deposits give a brown metachromasia and are birefringent when stained with cresyl violet (Hirsch and Peiffer, 1957). Hollander's technique stains sulphatide orange and is probably more specific for this lipid than cresyl violet (Pearse, 1972).

Protein histochemistry

The proteins of major interest in peripheral nerves are those associated with the myelin sheath lipids. Several techniques can be used to identify different classes of protein. They include labelled antibody techniques and acid—base 'histophysical' staining methods which depend in part upon the isoelectric point of the protein in unfixed cryostat sections (Adams, 1965). Histochemical techniques have been devised for various chemical groups such as the SS and SH groups of cystine and cysteine or for individual amino acids, e.g. the dimethylaminobenzaldehyde (DMAB) method for tryptophan (Adams, 1965; Pearse, 1968).

Myelin proteins can also be separated into two histochemical classes by treatment of the tissue with trypsin. (1) *Trypsin-resistant protein*. Following trypsin digestion a protein (neurokeratin) network remains in the myelin sheath; this protein is rich in tryptophan (Adams, 1965). (2) *Trypsin-digestible protein*. By comparing the staining reactions of untreated and trypsin digested nerve it is found that trypsin extracts a basic protein which is stained by anionic dyes such as trypan blue, amido black and phosphotungstic acid haematin (PTAH). Much of the myelin lipid is apparently attached to the basic protein component and it is these proteins that are lost from the sheath very early in the process of myelin breakdown (Hallpike, 1972). Furthermore, it is a part of the basic protein component of myelin which is encephalitogenic or neuritogenic in the induction of experimental allergic encephalomyelitis or neuritis (Leibowitz, 1972; Westall *et al.*, 1971).

Polysaccharide histochemistry

The complexity of polysaccharides and mucosubstances (mucopolysaccharides) has led to a reclassification both biochemically and histochemically (Pearse, 1968). With regard to the nervous system, the most important groups in Pearse's classification are as follows.

I. *Glycans* (polysaccharides or oligosaccharides)
    (a) *Homoglycans* (neutral polysaccharides: one monosaccharide component)
        Glycogen (contains glucose; PAS-positive; removed by diastase)
    (b) *Homopolyaminosaccharides*
        Chitin (contains *N*-acetyl-glucosamine)
    (c) *Heteroglycans* (two or more monosaccharide components) (acid mucopolysaccharides)
        (1) Glycosaminoglycans (PAS-negative)
            Sialoglycans (neuraminic acid) (heteropolyamino saccharides)
        (2) Glycosaminoglucuronoglycans (PAS-negative)
            Hyaluronic acid
            Chondroitin sulphates: A, B and C
            Heparin
II. *Polysaccharide–protein complexes*
        Chondroitin sulphate–protein
        Hyaluronic acid–protein
III. *Glycoproteins and glycopolypeptides*
        Serum glycoproteins (including PAS-positive immunoglobulins)
IV. *Glycolipids* (PAS-positive)
        Cerebrosides (hexose-containing sphingolipids)
        Gangliosides (hexose, hexosamine and neuraminic acid containing sphingolipids)
V.   *Glycolipid–protein complexes*
        Ox brain mucolipid
        Strandin (a complex polymer of ganglioside)

Acid mucopolysaccharides (AMPS) in the old nomenclature include the glycosaminoglycans (sialoglycans) and the glycosaminoglucuronoglycans (hyaluronic acid, chondroitin sulphates and heparin). They are found mainly in connective tissues, in certain body fluids and associated with the outer aspects of some membranes.

Fixation and staining reactions. Formalin is not regarded as a good fixative for mucosubstances, and better results are obtained with Carnoy's alcoholic–acetic acid fixative or by the use of cations from lead and barium salts (Adams, 1965). Quaternary ammonium compounds and dyes such as acridine orange have been used to precipitate and stain AMPS in tissues (Saunders, 1964). Glycogen can be retained in the tissue by using a variety of fixatives, including formalin, 80 per cent ethanol and Rossman's fluid, but much of the glycogen is lost unless Rossman's fluid is used for floating out and rehydrating paraffin sections (Swigart, Wagner and Atkinson, 1960).

Periodic acid–Schiff (PAS) method. Periodic acid reacts with hexose sugars in polysaccharides and oxidizes their adjacent 1,2-hydroxyl groups to aldehyde. Schiff's leucofuchsin reagent can then be used to form a red anil, azomethine or Schiff's base (Adams, 1965). Although the chemical mechanism of the PAS method is precise, various other hydroxyl groups (hydroxy-amine, hydroxy-keto, etc.) react, so that the technique cannot be used for direct identification of any one chemical substance in tissue sections. Despite this, it is a very useful method. Glycogen is PAS-positive and is extracted by diastase. Among the mucosubstances, homopolyaminosaccharides (neutral mucopolysaccharides; e.g. chitin), and a variety of mucoproteins, glycoproteins (e.g. gut mucins) and glycolipids are PAS-positive. Acid mucopolysaccharides are mainly PAS-negative (Adams, 1965).

Alcian blue. Alcian blue 8GS and later alcian blue 8GX have been used extensively in the histochemical localization of acid mucopolysaccharides. Identification of different groups of AMPS is achieved by: (a) staining at different pH; (b) staining at different concentrations of $MgCl_2$ (critical electrolyte concentration; CEC). (c) staining after enzyme digestion by testicular hyaluronidase or *Vibrio cholerae* neuraminidase.

(a) pH 2·5 (1 per cent alcian blue 8GX in 3 per cent acetic acid) stains weakly acidic sulphated mucosubstances, hyaluronic acid and sialoglycans dark blue. Strongly acidic sulphated mucins are stained only weakly or not at all. At pH 1·0 (1 per cent alcian blue 8GX in 0·1 N HCl) sulphated mucosubstances (chondroitin sulphates) are stained blue.

(b) *Critical electrolyte concentrations.* Sections are stained with alcian blue 8GX in 0·5 M sodium acetate buffer (pH 5·7) to which $MgCl_2$ has been added in concentrations varying from 0·1 M to 1·0 M. Hyaluronic acid, sialoglycans and some weakly acidic sulphomucins are *not stained* at or above a concentration of 0·1 M $MgCl_2$, whereas most sulphated mucosubstances stain strongly at 0·2 M $MgCl_2$. As a concentration of $MgCl_2$ rises, various mucosubstances fail to stain, but some epithelial mucins, cornea and mast cells are still alcianophilic at 1·0 M $MgCl_2$.

(c) *Differential extraction* of tissue sections by testicular hyaluronidase or *Vibrio cholerae* neuraminidase (Spicer and Warren, 1960) followed by alcian blue staining allows some differentiation between these two types of AMPS to be made. Similarly, protein-bound mucopolysaccharide is removed from tissue by trypsin digestion (Goodhead, 1957).

A combined alcian blue–PAS method stains mucosubstances either blue, pink or purple, depending upon their relative degrees of alcianophilia or PAS-reactivity.

Hale's colloidal iron technique. Metallic cations such as colloidal iron form salt linkages with anions of AMPS which can then be visualized by potassium ferricyanide as Prussian blue (Pearse, 1968). Strongly acidic mucopolysaccharides are stained blue by this technique. As the primary reaction product is in the form of electron-dense crystals, it can be used as an electron histochemical stain (Langley and Landon, 1968).

Mucosubstances in peripheral nerves. Acid mucopolysaccharides (glucosaminoglycans) are found in the axon, endoneurium and at the node of Ranvier (Langley and Landon, 1968), whereas little neutral or acid mucopolysaccharide is seen in myelin (Adams and Bayliss, 1968).

Enzyme histochemistry

There are now a large number of enzymes that can be stained histochemically. Many of these enzymes are associated with mitochondria and other cell organelles which are common to most cells. Enzyme techniques can be used to delineate Schwann cell cytoplasm and axoplasm. In the normal nerve there is little enzyme activity associated with the myelin sheath (Adams *et al.*, 1963b). The Schwann cytoplasm may be identified by mitochondrial enzymes such as succinic or lactic dehydrogenase, and NAD (NADH) tetrazolium reductase in either cryostat sections or teased fibres (Morgan-Hughes and Engel, 1968; Weller and Nester, 1972).

The enzymes associated with neural transmission in cholinergic nerves, viz. cholinesterases (Gomori, 1952; Pearse, 1972) allow the delineation of small non-myelinated fibres and muscle end-plates. Adrenergic nerves can be identified by the formalin-induced fluorescence (FIF) technique for catecholamines developed by Eränkö (1967) and Falck (1962). Several modifications are listed by Pearse (1972).

Many enzyme changes occur during Wallerian degeneration and segmental demyelination. There is an increase in the lysosomal hydrolytic enzymes associated with axon and myelin breakdown. Acid phosphatase is commonly used as a lysosomal marker, and can be detected in cryostat sections or teased preparations by the α-naphthyl phosphate and naphthol AS–TR phosphate methods and by the Gomori technique (Pearse, 1972). The advantage of the Gomori method is that the lead phosphate deposit is electron-dense and can be detected electron microscopically (see below).

The increase in proteolytic enzymes during myelin breakdown can be detected with the silver gelatin technique (Adams and Tuqan, 1961). Formalin-fixed cryostat sections are mounted on blackened photographic plate and incubated in either 0·15 M phosphate buffer (pH 7·6) or 0·15 M acetate buffer (pH 5·0) at 37 °C. The proteolytic enzymes in the sections remove the gelatin of the photographic plate and the silver grains it contains; enzyme activity is shown as clear zones on the plate (Hallpike, Adams and Bayliss, 1970).

21

Electron histochemistry

Various histochemical techniques have been adapted for electron microscopy (Pearse, 1972). Ideally, the reaction product should be electron-dense, discrete and accurately localized. With the use of lead salts as a final reaction product, various enzymes have been studied electron microscopically in normal and pathological nerves. They include acid phosphatase (Holtzman and Novikoff, 1965; Weller and Mellick, 1966; Weller and Herzog, 1970) and cholinesterase (Pearse, 1972). Mucosubstances (Langley and Landon, 1968) and phosphoglycerides (Weller *et al.*, 1965) have also been localized electron microscopically.

Histological measurements in sural nerve biopsies

The most useful measurements are obtained from teased fibre preparations and from transverse sections of epoxy resin-embedded nerve. Although not ideal, post-mortem specimens can also be used, especially for teased fibre studies. Various methods for quantification and their necessary precautions have been discussed by Dyck *et al.* (1968) and by Stevens, Lofgren and Dyck (1973).

(a) *Teased fibres*

The two most important measurements in teased fibres are the internodal length and the total diameter of myelinated nerve fibres. These can be measured over several internodes in single teased fibres by using an eye-piece graticule in the microscope. The results are plotted on a graph of length of the internode against fibre diameter; if each internode is plotted, the points from individual fibres can be joined together to show the range of internodal lengths (Lascelles and Thomas, 1966). In a normal fibre the internodal lengths are all approximately the same in any one fibre and are proportional to the diameter of that fibre (Stevens *et al.*, 1973). Groups of short internodes, or single short internodes along a fibre, are an indication of previous segmental demyelination and remyelination. If, on the other hand, all the internodes along a fibre are short, this suggests that axonal degeneration with subsequent regeneration has occurred sometime in the past.

In acute demyelinating neuropathies a widened nodal gap at the node of Ranvier is a very early stage in segmental demyelination which may be easily detected in individual teased fibres (Cavanagh and Jacobs, 1964; see Chapter 4).

(b) *Transverse sections*

One of the most difficult problems in the examination of biopsies of peripheral nerves is the detection of minor reductions in the number of nerve fibres. The density of nerve fibres within a fascicle can, however, be estimated by measuring the transverse area of a nerve fascicle and counting the number of nerve fibres within it. Pathological nerves can be compared with healthy controls. Large and small myelinated fibres are easily counted on enlarged photomicrographs of toluidine blue-stained epoxy resin sections. Non-myelinated fibres can be counted on similar photographs but more accurate estimates are obtained from electron micrographs. Myelinated fibre diameters and axon: myelin sheath ratios may also be measured on 1–2 μm epoxy resin sections, but care must be taken to avoid obliquely cut or artefactually damaged fibres (Dyck *et al.*, 1968). Various mechanical aids have been designed for measuring fibre diameters, including a Perspex disc with a central hole and concentric rings drawn at set distances from the centre. If the disc is placed over the fibre image, the mean diameter can be quickly estimated. Non-myelinated fibre diameters can only be measured accurately in electron micrographs. The histograms that can be constructed from these measurements are discussed in Chapter 3.

Artefact in peripheral nerve histology

Most of the artefacts in peripheral nerve histology result from crushing the fresh specimen or from poor preparation. Such artefacts are most prominent in epoxy resin-embedded material but may also be seen in paraffin sections and in teased preparations.

Crush artefact

The essentially liquid nature of the myelin sheath in peripheral nerves was recognized by Ranvier and by earlier workers. If a fresh nerve fibre is placed between a cover slip and a slide, distortion of the myelin sheath can be observed under the microscope when the nerve is compressed. Furthermore, if the nerve is placed in a hypotonic medium, the myelin swells and 'buds' from the cut end of the nerve in the form of spherules. Considerable distortion of enzyme staining patterns occurs if attempts are made to tease unfixed nerve fibres (Weller and Nester, 1972). Crush artefacts in nerve biopsies are probably due mainly to compression of the nerve by forceps or even by dabbing the nerve with a swab during surgical removal. Similar artefact may occur if the nerve is cut into small pieces before it is properly fixed. Histologically, the artefact may be gross and is usually seen most prominently in epoxy resin sections. Transverse sections of the nerve may show compressed, angulated fascicles and distortion of the large myelinated fibres (*Figure 4*). If the fresh nerve has been crushed, the axon and myelin sheath may be compressed into irregular globules along the nerve, or the axon may be extruded from the myelin sheath. This type of artefact may appear in transverse section as very thick myelin sheaths or distorted 'demyelinated' axons (*Figure 5*). Similar artefact can be detected in teased nerves.

Poor preparation

This may result in shrinkage of Schwann cell processes and axons together with splitting and disruption of myelin lamellae, especially in the thicker sheaths.

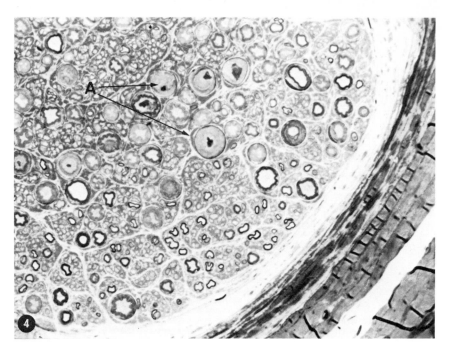

Fig. 4. Artefact *in a normal sural nerve: several large myelinated fibres in the fascicle are distorted (A). 1 µm Araldite section stained with toluidine blue.* × 482

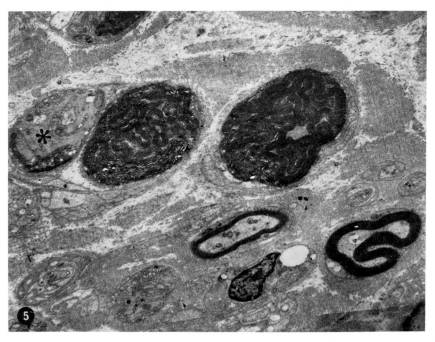

Fig. 5. Artefact *in peripheral nerve. An electron micrograph showing three distorted myelinated fibres; in one fibre (*) the axon has been extruded from the myelin sheath.* × 2455

24

Care must be taken to adjust the pH and osmolarity of the fixatives, particularly for electron microscopy.

MUSCLE BIOPSY IN PERIPHERAL NEUROPATHIES

Although it is often inadvisable to biopsy motor nerves directly, small intramuscular nerve bundles may be studied in muscle biopsies. Similarly, the terminal arborization of motor nerves and the motor end-plates on the muscle fibres may also be visualized. The secondary effects of denervation upon the muscle itself are also seen in muscle biopsies.

The muscle chosen for biopsy should be affected but not too severely, as it is difficult to interpret the changes in severely disorganized muscle. There are several muscle biopsy techniques for obtaining tissue for electron microscopy, histochemistry and paraffin embedding and for biochemical estimations (Weller, 1972; Dubowitz and Brooke, 1973). For this histological specimens there are three important considerations: prevention of artefactual trauma; prevention of excessive contraction of the muscle fibres during fixation; and the maintenance of the orientation of the muscle fibres, as it is easier to evaluate changes in an exact transverse or exact longitudinal sections than in a mixture of oblique cuts.

The muscle is exposed under local anaesthesia halfway between the origin and insertion; this is the region where nerves and the motor end-plates are usually situated. The sample for electron microscopy should be firmly held in a clamp to prevent contraction of the fibres when the specimen is plunged into glutaraldehyde fixative. Alternatively, a short length of sterile swab stick is placed upon the surface of the muscle parallel to the muscle fibres; then two atraumatic silk or catgut sutures are placed about 1 cm apart around the stick, biting about 1–2 mm into the muscle. The stick is cut free from the muscle, leaving a thin strand of muscle tissue clamped between the sutures to prevent contraction on contact with the fixative. A piece of tissue up to 2 cm long and 1 cm diameter is usually sufficient for histochemistry and paraffin embedding; this specimen is divided longitudinally into two pieces under a dissecting microscope. One portion is used for histochemistry and the other portion is placed upon a card in a damp atmosphere for about 15 min before it is placed in formalin; this short interval prevents excessive contraction as the muscle comes into contact with the fixative.

Histochemistry of muscle

There is less distortion and shrinkage of muscle fibres in cryostat sections than in paraffin-embedded material. In addition, enzyme activity within the muscle fibres allows differentiation of Type 1 (slow twitch) fibres and Type 2 (fast twitch) fibres.

A piece of muscle should be cut from the biopsy so that the orientation of the fibres is obvious. It is then plunged either into isopentane cooled by liquid nitrogen or straight into liquid nitrogen (−180 °C). Artefact may occur during the freezing due to ice crystal formation and the outer parts of the muscle specimen may show multiple holes in the fibres—the 'waffle artefact'. This can

TABLE 2

Histology and histochemistry of muscle

Histological features	Cryostat sections	Paraffin sections	Thick frozen fixed sections
Fibre typing	Myosin ATPase; NADH–TR; SDH	—	—
Fibre sizes	Myosin ATPase; diastase–PAS	Diastase–PAS	—
Phagocytosis	Haematoxylin and eosin (H. and E.) diastase–PAS	H. and E.; diastase–PAS	
Regeneration	H. and E.: trichrome	H. and E.; methyl green pyronin	—
Myelinated nerves	H. and E.; Sudan black B; diastase–PAS; trichrome	H. and E.; diastase–PAS; Loyez	Sudan black
Axons and nerve terminals	—	Glees and Marsland; Bodian; Palmgren	Schofield silver technique
Muscle end-plates	Cholinesterase	—	Cholinesterase
Vessels	H. and E.	Elastic stain (Verhoeff); H. and E.	—
Inflammatory cells	H. and E.	H. and E.; methyl green pyronin; PAS	—
Parasites	H. and E.; PAS	H. and E.; PAS	

be avoided by rolling the muscle in starch glove powder before plunging it quickly into liquid nitrogen. The specimen is removed from the liquid nitrogen when it stops bubbling (30–60 s) and is then quickly placed in a small container pre-cooled in the cryostat (–20 °C) in the bottom of which is a piece of frozen, dampened cotton-wool. In this way the muscle can either be stored at –20 °C or allowed to reach cryostat temperature and then cut. The block is easily trimmed with a scalpel and orientated for exact transverse sectioning. Attachment to the chuck is achieved by placing a small drop of gum acacia on a chuck cooled to –20 °C and pressing the block into the gum just as it freezes.

Apart from histological stains (haematoxylin and eosin, trichrome, Van Gieson), serial sections are stained by enzyme techniques (myosin ATPase, NAD (NADH)–tetrazolium reductase, myophosphorylase, succinic dehydrogenase) which differentiate Type 1 and Type 2 fibres Dubowitz and Brooke (1973). Diastase–PAS is a very useful technique, as it stains the thin sheath of endomysial connective tissue and thus outlines the fibres; any size disparity is quickly apparent. Some of the techniques used in the study of muscle biopsy are summarized in *Table 2*.

Histology of nerves in muscle biopsies

Muscle biopsy presents an opportunity to study motor nerve fibres and their endings. The myelinated nerves are well visualized in diastase–PAS-stained cryostat or paraffin sections of muscle. Greater lengths of nerve can be studied in thick (50 μm) frozen sections of fixed muscle stained with Sudan black for myelinated fibres (Cavanagh, Passingham and Vogt, 1964) or by Schofield's silver method for axons and their terminal arborizations (Drury and Wallington, 1967). Muscle end-plates can be visualized by cholinesterase staining (Pearse, 1972). Intravital staining of nerve terminals with methylene blue can also be used to study human biopsies (Coërs, Telerman-Toppet and Gérard, 1973).

REFERENCES

Adams, C. W. M. (1961). 'The perchloric acid–naphthoquinone method for the histochemical localisation of cholesterol.' *Nature (London)*, **192**, 331.

Adams, C. W. M. (1965). In *Neurohistochemistry*. Amsterdam; Elsevier.

Adams, C. W. M., Abdulla, Y. H., Bayliss, O. B. and Weller, R. O. (1966). 'Histochemical detection of triglyceride esters with specific lipases and a calcium–lead sulphide technique.' *J. Histochem. Cytochem.*, **14**, 385.

Adams, C. W. M. and Bayliss, O. B. (1968). 'Histochemistry of myelin. VII. Analysis of lipid–protein relationships and the absence of acid mucopolysaccharide.' *J. Histochem. Cytochem.*, **16**, 110.

Adams, C. W. M. and Bayliss, O. B., (1975). 'Lipid histochemistry.' In *Techniques of Biochemical and Biophysical Morphology*, Vol. 2. Ed. by D. Glick and R. Rosenbaum. New York; Wiley.

Adams, C. W. M., Bayliss, O. B. and Ibrahim, M. Z. M. (1963a). 'Modifications to histochemical methods for phosphoglyceride and cerebroside.' *J. Histochem. Cytochem.*, **11**, 560.

Adams, C. W. M., Davison, A. N. and Gregson, N. A. (1963b). 'Enzyme inactivity of myelin: histochemical and biochemical evidence.' *J. Neurochem.*, **10**, 383.

REFERENCES

Adams, C. W. M. and Tuqan, N. A. (1961). 'Histochemistry of myelin. II. Proteins, lipid–protein dissociation and proteinase activity in Wallerian degeneration.' *J. Neurochem.,* **6**, 334.

Bearn, A. G. (1972). 'Cell culture in inherited disease with some notes on genetic heterogeneity.' *N. Engl. J. Med.,* **286**, 764–767.

Bodian, M. and Lake, B. D. (1963). 'The rectal approach to neuropathology.' *Br. J. Surg.,* **50**, 702.

Cavanagh, J. B. and Jacobs, J. M. (1964). 'Some quantitative aspects of diphtheritic neuropathy.' *Br. J. Exp. Pathol.,* **45**, 309.

Cavanagh, J. B., Passingham, R. J. and Vogt, J. A. (1964). 'Staining of sensory and motor nerves in muscles with Sudan black B.' *J. Pathol. Bacteriol.,* **88**, 89.

Coërs, C., Telerman-Toppet, N. and Gérard, J.-M. (1973). 'Terminal innervation ratio in neuromuscular disease. I. Methods and controls.' *Arch. Neurol.,* **29**, 210.

Drury, R. A. B. and Wallington, E. A. (1967). In *Carleton's Histochemical Technique,* 4th edn. London; Oxford University Press.

Dubowitz, V. and Brooke, M. H. (1973). In *Muscle Biopsy: A Modern Approach.* London; Saunders.

Dyck, P. J., Conn, D. L. and Okazaki, H. (1972). 'Necrotizing angiopathic neuropathy. Three-dimensional morphology of fiber degeneration related to sites of occluded vessels.' *Mayo Clin. Proc.,* **47**, 461.

Dyck, P. J., Gutrecht, J. A., Bastron, J. A., Karnes, W. E. and Dale, A. J. D. (1968). 'Histological and teased-fiber measurements of sural nerve in disorders of lower motor and primary sensory neurones.' *Mayo Clin. Proc.,* **43**, 81.

Dyck, P. J. and Lofgren, E. P. (1966). 'Method of fascicular biopsy of human peripheral nerve for electrophysiologic and histologic study.' *Mayo Clin. Proc.,* **41**, 778.

Eränkö, O. (1967). 'The practical histochemical demonstration of catecholamines by formaldehyde-induced fluorescence.' *J. Roy Microscop. Soc.,* **87**, 259.

Falck, B. (1962). 'Observations on the possibilities of the cellular localisation of monoamines by a fluorescence method.' *Acta Physiol. Scand.,* **56**, Suppl. **197**, 1.

Gallyas, F. (1963). 'The histochemical identification of phosphoglycerides in myelin.' *J. Neurochem.,* **10**, 125.

Glauert, A. M. (1975). In *Fixation, Dehydration and Embedding of Biological Specimens.* Amsterdam; North-Holland.

Gomori, G. (1952). In *Microscopic Histochemistry,* p. 189. Chicago; University of Chicago Press.

Goodhead, B. (1957). 'The development of a ground substance in the cerebral cortex of the rat.' *Acta Anat.,* **29**, 297.

Hallpike, J. F. (1972). 'Enzyme and protein changes in myelin breakdown and multiple sclerosis.' *Progr. Histochem. Cytochem.,* **3**, 179.

Hallpike, J. F., Adams, C. W. M. and Bayliss, O. B. (1970). 'Histochemistry of myelin IX neutral and acid proteinases in early Wallerian degeneration.' *Histochem. J.,* **2**, 209.

Hayat, M. A. (1970). *Principles and Techniques of Electron Microscopy: Biological Applications,* Vol. I. New York; Van Nostrand Reinhold.

Hirsch, T. and Peiffer, J. (1957). In *Cerebral Lipidoses.* Ed. by J. N. Cummings. Oxford.

Holtzman, E. and Novikoff, A. B. (1965). 'Lysosomes in the rat sciatic nerve following crush.' *J. Cell Biol.,* **27**, 651.

Jacobs, J. (1967). 'Experimental diphtheritic neuropathy in the rat.' *Br. J. Exp. Pathol.,* **48**, 204.

Kalyanaraman, U. P. and Finlayson, M. H. (1969). 'Microdissection in enzyme histochemistry of peripheral nerve.' *J. Neurol. Sci.,* **9**, 77.

Langley, O. K. and Landon, D. N. (1968). 'A light and electron histochemical approach to the node of Ranvier and myelin of peripheral nerve fibres.' *J. Histochem. Cytochem.,* **15**, 722.

Lascelles, R. G. and Thomas, P. K. (1966). 'Changes due to age in internodal length in the sural nerve in man.' *J. Neurol. Neurosurg. Psychiat.,* **29**, 40.

Leibowitz, S. (1972). 'Immunology of multiple sclerosis.' In *Research on Multiple Sclerosis,* pp. 149–168. Ed. by C. W. M. Adams. Springfield, Illinois; Charles C. Thomas.

Lewis, P. R. and Lobban, M. C. (1961). 'Chemical specificity of the Schultz test for steroids.' *J. Histochem. Cytochem.,* **9**, 2.

Morgan-Hughes, J. A. and Engel, W. K. (1968). 'Histochemical patterns in single peripheral nerve fibers.' *Arch. Neurol.,* **19**, 613.

Ochoa, J. and Mair, W. G. P. (1969). 'The normal sural nerve in man. II. Changes in the axons and Schwann cells due to aging.' *Acta Neuropath. (Berlin),* **13**, 217.

REFERENCES

Pearse, A. G. E. (1968). In *Histochemistry—Theoretical and Applied,* 3rd edn, Vol 1. London; Churchill.

Pearse, A. G. E. (1972). In *Histochemistry—Theoretical and Applied,* 3rd edn, Vol. 2. Edinburgh; Churchill Livingstone.

Saunders, A. M. (1964). 'Histochemical identification of acid mucopolysaccharides with Acridine Orange.' *J. Histochem. Cytochem.,* **12,** 164.

Spicer, S. S. and Warren, L. (1960). 'The histochemistry of sialic acid containing mucoproteins.' *J. Histochem. Cytochem.,* **8,** 135.

Stevens, J. C., Lofgren, E. P. and Dyck, P. J. (1973). 'Histometric evaluation of branches of peroneal nerve: technique for combined biopsy of muscle nerve and cutaneous nerve.' *Brain Res.,* **52,** 37.

Swigart, R. H., Wagner, C. E. and Atkinson, W. B. (1960). 'The preservation of glycogen in fixed tissues and tissue sections.' *J. Histochem. Cytochem.,* **8,** 74.

Weller, R. O. (1972). 'Histopathological techniques in the investigation of muscle disease.' *Proc. Roy. Soc. Med.,* **65,** 615.

Weller, R. O., Bayliss, O. B., Abdulla, Y. H. and Adams, C. W. M. (1965). 'The electron-histochemical demonstration of phosphoglyceride.' *J. Histochem. Cytochem.,* **13,** 690.

Weller, R. O. and Herzog, I. (1970). 'Schwann cell lysosomes in hypertrophic neuropathy and in normal human nerves.' *Brain,* **93,** 347.

Weller, R. O. and Mellick, R. S. (1966). 'Acid phosphatase and lysosome activity in diphtheritic neuropathy and Wallerian degeneration.' *Br. J. Exp. Pathol.,* **47,** 425.

Weller, R. O. and Nester, B. (1972). 'Early changes at the node of Ranvier in segmental demyelination: histochemical and electron microscopic observations.' *Brain,* **95,** 665.

Westall, F. C., Robinson, A. B., Caccam, J., Jackson, J. and Eylar, E. H. (1971). 'Essential chemical requirements for induction of allergic encephalomyelitis.' *Nature (London),* **229,** 22.

3

Normal Peripheral Nerves

Peripheral nerves arise from the spinal cord and include all but the first two pairs of cranial nerves (*Gray's Anatomy:* Warwick and Williams, 1973). They contain axons from several different types of neurone serving various effector organs or sensory endings. Motor fibres from anterior horn cells in the spinal cord are the main neural components of the anterior spinal roots, but preganglionic sympathetic and parasympathetic fibres are also present at certain levels. The posterior roots contain sensory fibres whose cell bodies are in the posterior root ganglia. As the spinal roots fuse, mixed nerve trunks are formed. Plexuses of nerves are found in the lower cervical and lumbosacral regions. It is from these plexuses that the major nerve trunks form and carry a mixture of motor and sensory nerve fibres to supply the upper and lower limbs. The major sympathetic outflow is in the thoracic region, where preganglionic myelinated fibres from neurones in the lateral horns of grey matter in the spinal cord pass out in the anterior roots to the paravertebral chain of sympathetic ganglia, or into the splanchnic nerves. Similarly, the preganglionic parasympathetic fibres pass out in the anterior spinal roots in the pelvic region and in the third, ninth and tenth cranial nerves. The parasympathetic ganglia are situated in, or near, their effector organs.

Many of the major spinal nerves, including those in the limbs, run in close association with arteries and veins (neurovascular bundles). Towards the periphery, however, the nerves are associated with veins; this applies particularly to the superficial sensory nerves. Accounts of the anatomical distribution of peripheral nerves and autonomic plexuses throughout the body are given in standard anatomy (*Gray's Anatomy*) and neurological texts (Brain and Walton, 1969).

DEVELOPMENT OF PERIPHERAL NERVES

The nerve fibres of the anterior spinal roots grow out from neuroblasts in the anterior and lateral parts of the mantle layer of the developing spinal cord in the fourth to sixth week of intra-uterine life. They penetrate the overlying marginal layer and grow into the myotomes of the appropriate mesodermal somites. As the limb buds begin to appear at the end of the fourth week, the ventral rami grow into the developing musculature.

Sensory nerve fibres develop as outgrowths from the cells of the spinal ganglia which are derived from the neural crest. As the neural tube closes posteriorly, the lips of the neural fold fuse to form the neural crest, which then separates to form oval-shaped masses of cells on each side of the primitive spinal cord. Some of the neuroblasts in the neural crest tissue develop into sensory posterior root ganglion cells, whereas others, from the anterior part, form sympathetic ganglion cells and chromaffin cells. Schwann cells and ganglion satellite cells also develop from spongioblasts of the neural crest.

Two neurites arise from each sensory ganglion cell, so that a bipolar neurone is formed. One process grows centrally into the spinal cord to form the posterior spinal root and the other process grows peripherally to mingle with the fibres of the anterior root to form a mixed spinal nerve. As development proceeds, the ganglion cell becomes round and the central and peripheral processes fuse to form a single stem; the cell is thus converted to a unipolar neurone.

Apart from the olfactory and optic nerves, the cranial nerves develop in a similar way to the spinal nerves. The oculomotor, trochlear, abducent and hypoglossal nerves supply somite-derived ocular and tongue muscles, whereas the motor fibres in the trigeminal, facial, glossopharyngeal and vagus nerves supply striated muscle derived from branchial arches. The neurone cell bodies of these nerves are situated near the mid-line in the brain stem. A neural crest forms in the region of the hind-brain and mid-brain, and it is homologous with the neural crest of the spinal cord. The ganglia of the vagus, glossopharyngeal, facial and trigeminal nerves and part of the vestibulocochlear ganglion develop from the neural crest. In addition, sympathetic and parasympathetic ganglia develop from neural crest elements associated with the cranial nerves. There is some evidence that the enteric ganglia in the walls of the gut develop from both vagal neural crest and spinal neural crest (Andrew, 1971).

There is close interdependence of neural and mesodermal structures during development; if the limb nerves fail to grow, the mesodermal structures do not develop. Similarly, if there is disturbance of the normal segmentation of mesodermal structures, corresponding abnormalities are seen in the neural structures. No adequate hypothesis has yet been advanced, however, to explain how the developing neural processes make contact with the relevant muscle cells or sensory end-organs. The involvement of chemical mediators has been postulated and various 'nerve growth factors' have been extracted from a number of tissues (Levi-Montalcini and Angeletti, 1968). Administration of anti-nerve growth factor antibodies to foetuses will block the development of the sympathetic nervous system but has little effect on somatic motor or sensory nerves (Aguayo, Martin and Bray, 1972).

MOTOR NEURONES

The neurone cell bodies that innervate skeletal muscle and the branchial arch musculature in the cranial region are situated in the anterior horns of grey matter in the spinal cord and its homologues in the brain stem (Brodal, 1969). Enlargements of the cord in the cervical and lumbar segments mark the major regions supplying the upper and lower limbs.

Many of the anterior horn cells are large motor neurones with vesicular nuclei and prominent nucleoli (*Figure 31*). The cytoplasm contains clumps of 'Nissl substance', which consists of cisternae of rough surface endoplasmic reticulum and clumps of polyribosomes (RNA) usually associated with protein synthesis. The axon, however, contains relatively little RNA. Although the cell body of the neurone may be 100 µm in diameter, the axon arising from it may be more than 1 m in length and 8–10 µm in diameter. Most of the cytoplasm of the cell, and most of the cell surface membrane, therefore, is contained in the axon.

SENSORY NEURONES

The first sensory neurones are situated in the posterior root ganglia or the corresponding ganglia in the cranial region. In the spinal region the posterior root sensory ganglia are just proximal to the fusion of the anterior and posterior roots. Each ganglion contains almost spherical neurones surrounded by satellite cells (*Figure 6*). They are unipolar neurones and their central processes pass into the spinal cord, either directly into the ipsilateral ascending dorsal columns or they synapse with other neurones in the cord, whose axons

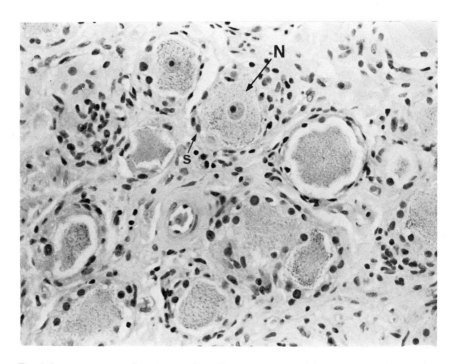

Fig. 6. Posterior root ganglion. Large spherical sensory neurones (N) are surrounded by satellite cells (s). H. and E. stain; × 300

then ascend mainly in the spinocerebellar and spinothalamic pathways. All afferents branch, giving segmental innervation as well as ascending tracts.

THE AUTONOMIC NERVOUS SYSTEM

The autonomic nervous system is under the control of centres in the brain, many of which are in the hypothalamus. Autonomic nerves innervate smooth muscle in many visceral blood vessels and many of the secretory glands. The sympathetic part of the system is concerned mainly with preparation for violent activity, often described as 'fight or flight', whereas the parasympathetic part is connected more with anabolic, excretory and reproductive activities. In both the sympathetic and parasympathetic systems preganglionic fibres run from the central nervous system to peripheral ganglia; postganglionic fibres pass from the ganglion cells to the organs which they innervate. Most postganglionic sympathetic fibres are adrenergic and release catecholamine neural transmitters at their nerve terminals. Sympathetic nerves innervating sweat glands appear to be an exception; they are cholinergic and release acetyl choline at their nerve terminals. Parasympathetic nerves are also cholinergic.

The sympathetic and parasympathetic systems have separate outflow pathways from the brain and spinal cord. Preganglionic neurones of the sympathetic system are situated in the lateral horns of grey matter in the thoracic spinal cord, and their myelinated nerves pass out in the ventral spinal roots of all the thoracic segments and the first lumbar segment. Most of the fibres pass into the sympathetic chain which runs either side of the vertebral bodies from the cervical region to the coccygeal region. There are three cervical, eleven thoracic, four lumbar, four sacral and one coccygeal ganglia in the chain, connected by trunks of nerves. Although the outflow of sympathetic preganglionic fibres is restricted to the thoracic and first lumbar segments of the spinal cord, the preganglionic fibres pass up and down the sympathetic chain to synapse with the ganglion cells at other levels. In addition, sympathetic fibres pass through the chain into more peripheral ganglia (e.g. coeliac ganglia) and into sympathetic plexuses via such routes as the splanchnic nerves. Non-myelinated postganglionic fibres arising from the neurones in the sympathetic chain pass back into the spinal nerves and are distributed to blood vessels and various viscera. Postganglionic fibres from peripheral ganglia may pass into nerve plexuses and thence to the viscera.

The normal growth and differentiation of sympathetic ganglia in the foetus depend upon a specific protein, nerve growth factor, which is found in many tissues but, for some unknown reason, is abundant in the salivary glands of male mice (Levi-Montalcini and Angeletti, 1968). Nerve growth factor also induces an increase in the enzymes tyrosine hydroxylase and dopamine β-hydroxylase which are concerned with the synthesis of catecholamines (Thoenen, 1972). Administration of an antiserum to nerve growth factor to developing animals retards or prevents the normal development of the sympathetic nervous system (Aguayo *et al.*, 1972).

The outflow of preganglionic parasympathetic fibres is confined to the cranial and sacral regions. Unlike the sympathetic nerve system, the parasympathetic ganglion cells are situated very close to the viscera which they innervate. In the cranial region the principal parasympathetic outflow is in the third, seventh, ninth and tenth nerves. Many of the postganglionic fibres arise from ganglia in the head region; the vagus nerve, however, supplies much of the gut, where the majority of the postganglionic fibres arise from small groups of neurones within the viscera that they supply. The sacral parasympathetic preganglionic fibres arise from the second and third sacral segments and pass into the vesical plexus.

Afferent fibres that subserve the sympathetic system are both myelinated and non-myelinated; they enter the central nervous system through the posterior spinal roots at all levels and their neurone cell bodies are in the posterior root ganglia. The principal parasympathetic afferents have their neurone cell bodies in the inferior ganglion of the vagus and pass into the central nervous system with that nerve.

MORPHOLOGY OF NORMAL PERIPHERAL NERVE

Naked eye inspection of a normal peripheral nerve reveals a white cord-like structure with a fairly smooth surface but usually with some loose adipose tissue adhering to it. Many large fasciculi are seen in major peripheral nerves such as the sciatic, but towards the periphery, where the nerve branches extensively, it is composed of many smaller fasciculi. Medium-sized nerves, e.g. femoral and median nerves, are often closely bound to arteries and veins in neurovascular bundles.

Epineurium

Transverse histological sections of a nerve reveal an outer connective tissue sheath, the epineurium, which binds the nerve fascicles together (*Figure 7*). It is composed of loose fibrous tissue with some adipose tissue. In most nerves of moderate size, such as the sural nerve, the main single muscular artery runs longitudinally along the nerve within the epineurium, accompanied by smaller branches, veins and lymphatics. The main artery receives anastomotic branches along its length; elimination of these regional sources of supply may cause ischaemic damage within the nerve (Adams, 1943).

Perineurium

Each nerve fascicle is surrounded by a perineurial sheath composed of concentric layers of flattened cells separated by layers of collagen. The number of cell layers varies, depending upon the size of the nerve fascicle. In the sural nerve some eight layers may be seen, but there is a gradual reduction in thickness of the perineurium as the nerve branches become smaller.

Electron microscopy shows that each thin cellular lamella is surrounded by a basement membrane which separates it from the parallel bundles of collagen aligned parallel to the long axis of the nerve fascicle (*Figure 8*). In man the basement membrane is thicker than in smaller mammals. There are junctional complexes (zonulae occludentes) (Farquhar and Palade, 1963) between the

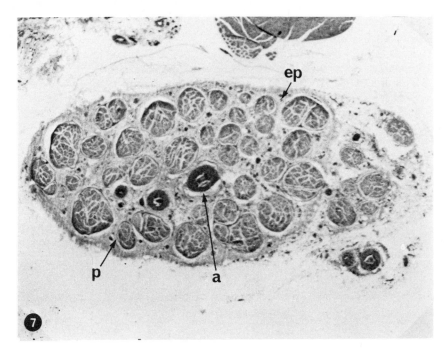

Fig. 7. *Transverse section of a peripheral nerve containing several nerve fascicles. Epineurium (ep); epineurial arteries (a); perineurium (p). H. and E. stain; × 16*

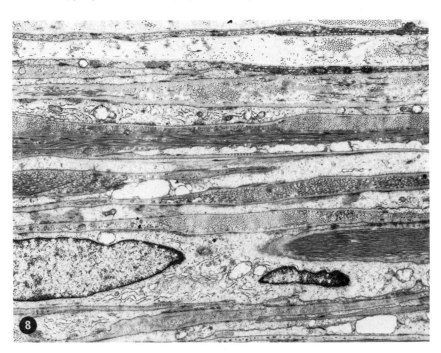

Fig. 8. *Electron micrograph of perineurium. Thin cell lamellae are separated by bundles of collagen fibres. × 6650*

cells within each layer and many pinocytotic vesicles are seen within the cells. The cells only broaden in the perinuclear region. Permeability studies with isotope-labelled proteins and with fluorescent-labelled proteins (Olsson, 1968) suggest that the perineurium is a very significant permeability barrier. Material injected into the nerve fascicle tends to travel longitudinally along the fascicle, whereas substances of large molecular weight injected around the nerve permeate the perineurium very poorly. When the perineurium is separated from the nerve and stretched flat, its structure as a cellular sheet is more apparent. In the nerve roots the perineurium is replaced by layers of arachnoid cells (Gamble and Eames, 1966).

Endoneurium

This is the compartment enclosed by the perineurial sheath. It contains the nerve fibres, Schwann cells and blood vessels together with bundles of endoneurial collagen fibres orientated longitudinally along the nerve fascicle. Thin cellular septa traverse the larger fascicles, breaking the endoneurium into smaller segments. Fibroblasts are also found in the endoneurium and moderate numbers of mast cells are seen in the nerve fascicle in many species, including man (*Figure 9*) (Olsson, 1971). The spaces between the collagen fibres and cellular components are filled with acid mucopolysaccharides (glucosaminoglycans) (Langley and Landon, 1968). Cylindrical, hyaline bodies—Renaut bodies—occur in the endoneurial compartment; they are composed of randomly orientated collagen fibres, glucosaminoglycans and spidery cells resembling fibroblasts (Asbury, 1973). Their significance is not known but they may cause some confusion to the unwary observer.

When single myelinated nerve fibres are teased from a nerve fascicle, endoneurial collagen adheres to the surface. Early descriptions laid some stress upon this phenomenon; the outer endoneurial sheath (of Plenk and Laidlaw) was distinguished from the endoneurial sheath that more closely enveloped each myelinated nerve fibre (the sheath of Key and Retzius). Electron microscope studies have shown that both these sheaths consist of collagen fibrils. In the outer sheath the fibrils are arranged in parallel bundles, but close to the Schwann cell basement membrane the collagen fibres are often small and more randomly arranged; the innermost sheath together with the basement membrane stains as reticulin. Not all species show a distinct demarcation between the different layers of the endoneurium. Very little differentiation is seen in man, but the rabbit nerve shows a progressive increase in the thickness of the collagen fibres from the fine endoneurial fibres to the coarse fibres in the perineurium (Thomas, 1963).

The endoneurial compartment extends the length of the nerve, proximally into the roots and distally until the perineurial sheath is lost from the very fine branches. Less collagen is seen in the endoneurium of the roots compared with the main peripheral nerve trunks; this may be the reason why spinal root nerve fibres are less easily separated from one another by teasing (Gamble and Eames, 1964).

Dyes or labelled material injected under slight pressure into the nerve trunks tend to flow easily along the endoneurial compartment and may enter the subarachnoid space proximally. Although nutrients almost certainly diffuse

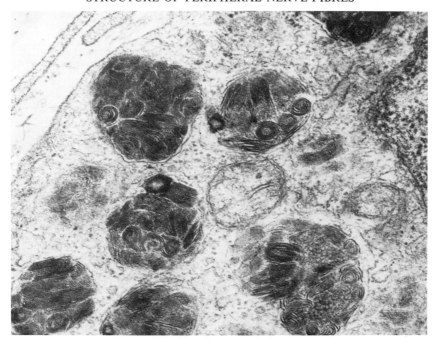

Fig. 9. Mast cell granules in a human peripheral nerve showing typical scroll-like ultrastructure. Electron micrograph × 5550

through the endoneurial connective tissue from the endoneurial blood vessels to the Schwann cells and nerve fibres, the environment appears to be rigidly controlled by the blood–nerve barrier, which does not allow extraneous protein-bound material either through the blood vessels or through the perineurium.

The longitudinal orientation of the endoneurial collagen appears to play an important role in minimizing the stretching of peripheral nerves but allowing them to bend as the limbs flex. It is possible also that the collagenous framework plays some role in maintaining pathways for regeneration of peripheral nerves.

STRUCTURE OF PERIPHERAL NERVE FIBRES

Most peripheral nerves contain myelinated and non-myelinated fibres. Some autonomic nerves, however, contain very few myelinated fibres; among these, the most extensively studied examples are the abdominal vagus in the rabbit (King and Thomas, 1971) and the cervical sympathetic trunk in the rat (Dyck and Hopkins, 1972). Both types of fibre can be seen in 1 μm Araldite sections of peripheral nerve when stained with toluidine blue (*Figure 10*) or viewed under phase contrast, but non-myelinated fibres are best demonstrated by electron microscopy. Myelinated fibres can be demonstrated in paraffin sections (*Figure 11*), especially if stained for myelin by Luxol fast blue, Loyez

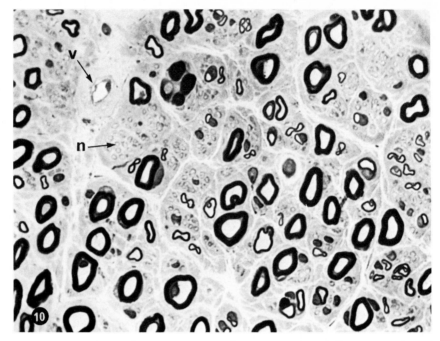

Fig. 10. T.S. sural nerve showing large and small diameter myelinated fibres. Non-myelinated axons (n). Endoneurial blood vessel (v). 1 μm section stained with toluidine blue. × 788

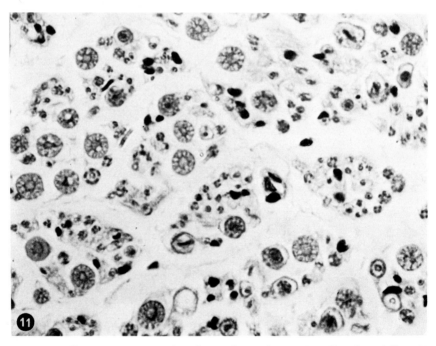

Fig. 11. Paraffin transverse section of sural nerve showing large and small myelinated fibres. H. and E. stain; × 788

or Heidenhain's haematoxylin techniques. Frozen sections stained with Sudan black or viewed in polarized light are also useful for myelinated fibres.

Non-myelinated axons are difficult to visualize satisfactorily in paraffin transverse sections of nerve, but the axons can be stained by silver techniques (Palmgren, Glees and Marsland, Bodian) and followed in longitudinal sections. Small nerve branches in various viscera such as stomach or large and small bowel contain many non-myelinated fibres which can be demonstrated either by silver methods (Fraher, 1972) or acetyl cholinesterase stains.

COMPOSITION OF PERIPHERAL NERVES

Not all peripheral nerves have the same composition of myelinated and non-myelinated fibres. The diameter of the axon and myelin sheath may vary even in a single nerve fibre from one anatomical site to another. Williams and Wendell-Smith (1971) calculated, for example, that cross-sectional areas of motor axons in the nerve supplying the rabbit gastrocnemius muscle are reduced by 25 per cent when compared with the same fibres in the ventral root. On the other hand, the myelin sheaths for any particular axon diameter are thicker in the nerve to gastrocnemius than in either the ventral spinal root or the sural nerve.

Most biopsies of peripheral nerve in human patients are taken from the sural nerve at the ankle and it is the composition of this nerve that has been most thoroughly studied. Ochoa and Mair (1969a) studied the transverse sections of sural nerve biopsies from seven normal individuals aged between 15 and 59 years of age. Using a combination of 1 μm thick Araldite sections stained with toluidine blue and electron microscopy, they found that 90 per cent of the cell nuclei in the endoneurial compartment of the nerve belonged to Schwann cells; the rest of the cells were mainly fibroblasts and capillary endothelium. Occasional mast cells are also present in the endoneurium. Eighty per cent of the Schwann cells are associated with non-myelinated axons. The non-myelinated fibres are nearly four times as numerous (approximately 30 000 per square millimetre of nerve) as the myelinated fibres (average 8000 per square millimetre). Histograms of fibre diameters (*Figure 12*) show that non-myelinated axons have a range of 0·5–3·0 μm in a unimodal distribution; a bimodal distribution is seen in older subjects (Ochoa and Mair, 1969b).

Myelinated fibres have a range of external diameter (axon plus myelin sheath) of 2–17 μm and show a bimodal distribution with peaks at 5 μm and 13 μm (*Figure 13*). Such a bimodal distribution with populations of small- and large-diameter myelinated fibres can easily be seen in a transverse section of normal sural nerve (*Figure 10*).

When axon diameters of non-myelinated and myelinated fibres are compared, there is little overlap in either man (Ochoa and Mair, 1969a) or rat (Weller and Das Gupta, 1968). This feature is very useful for deciding whether an axon that has no myelin sheath is truly non-myelinated or whether it has become demyelinated (see Chapter 4). Most histologically normal axons over 3 μm in diameter should have a myelin sheath unless the axon is cut transversely through the centre of a node of Ranvier. There is a correlation between the axon diameter and myelin sheath thickness. If the axon diameter (d) is plotted against $2 \times$ the myelin sheath thickness (m) (i.e. $2m =$ total fibre

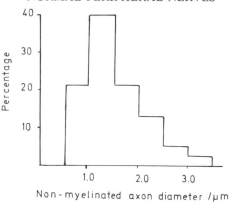

Fig. 12. Histogram showing size distribution of non-myelinated fibres in a normal adult sural nerve (courtesy of J. Neurol. Neurosurg. Pyschiat.)

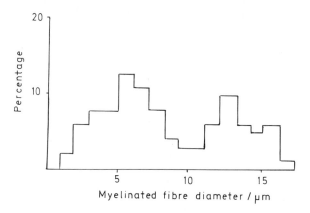

Fig. 13. Histogram to show the fibre spectrum of myelinated nerve fibres in an adult human sural nerve

diameter − d), there is a rectilinear correlation with the thicker sheaths surrounding the larger axons. A straight-line relationship is seen in both mature and immature nerves (Williams and Wendell-Smith, 1971). Physiologically, the important relationship is between axon diameter and total fibre diameter. A value of 0·6 for this ratio is the theoretical optimum for conduction in myelinated fibres (Rushton, 1951), but this is attained only in the larger-diameter fibres (Williams and Wendell-Smith, 1971).

Internodal lengths in normal teased nerve bear a variable positive correlation to total fibre diameter but they also vary according to local growth patterns (Vizoso and Young, 1948). In general, within the same nerve, the larger-diameter fibres have longer internodal lengths and this is reasonably constant within short lengths of the same nerve fibre. This correlation is disturbed in the sural nerves of older patients (Lascelles and Thomas, 1966), presumably owing to previous axonal degeneration and regeneration or segmental demyelination and subsequent remyelination (see Chapter 4).

CONDUCTION OF NERVE IMPULSES
CLASSIFICATION OF PERIPHERAL NERVE FIBRES

The classification of peripheral nerve fibres is based mainly on the total diameter of the fibre, i.e. axon and the myelin sheath, if it is present (Warwick and Williams, 1973). Larger-diameter myelinated nerve fibres conduct at a faster rate than small myelinated and non-myelinated fibres, so the classification also relates to functional conduction velocities.

Class A fibres are somatic afferent and efferent myelinated nerve fibres.
Class B fibres are myelinated preganglionic autonomic fibres.
Class C fibres are non-myelinated autonomic and sensory fibres.

Each class is subdivided partly on a functional basis and partly on size and conduction velocity (Boyd and Davey, 1968; Paintal, 1973).

Afferent (sensory) fibres in Class A (myelinated fibres)

Group I: up to 20 μm diameter with a conduction velocity about 100 m s^{-1}. Fibres in this group carry impulses from muscle spindles (intrafusal muscle fibres) and tendon organs.
Group II: 5–15 μm diameter with a conduction velocity of 20–90 m s^{-1}. These fibres carry impulses from mechanoreceptors and secondary endings on muscle spindles (intrafusal muscle fibres).
Group III: 1–7 μm diameter conducting at 12–30 m s^{-1}. They supply hair receptors and blood vessels. Some *pain* sensation is also a function of fibres in this group.

Efferent (motor) fibres in Class A (myelinated fibres)

α: Up to 17 μm diameter fibres conducting at 50–100 m s^{-1}. They supply the extrafusal striated muscle fibres; the fast twitch (Type 2) fibres more than the slow twitch (Type 1) fibres.
β: fibres supplying slow twitch (Type 1) muscle fibres and the intrafusal fibres (muscle spindles).
γ: 2–10 μm diameter conducting at 10–45 m s^{-1} and supplying intrafusal fibres (muscle spindles).

Class B fibres (myelinated preganglionic autonomic fibres)

These nerve fibres are small, 3 μm diameter, and conduct impulses at 3–15 m s^{-1}.

Class C fibres (non-myelinated fibres)

0·2–1·5 μm in diameter, conducting at 0·3–1·6 m s^{-1}. This class is composed of postganglionic autonomic and afferent fibres, including pain fibres.

CONDUCTION OF NERVE IMPULSES

In the resting state there is a difference in electrical potential across the neuronal and thus the axonal cell membrane. The inside of the cell has a net negative charge of 70–100 mV with respect to the interstitial fluid outside the cell. This potential is maintained by difference in ion concentrations between the inside of the cell and the interstitial fluid. Potassium and protein are the major ions inside the cell, whereas sodium and chloride ions have a higher concentration in the interstitial fluid; sodium is continually diffusing into the cell and potassium tends to pass out of the cell. The differential sodium–potassium concentrations are maintained in the resting cell by energy-dependent pumping mechanisms and at equilibrium there is a slightly lower positive ion concentration inside the cell than outside, which results in the negative intracellular charge. Calcium ions contribute to the maintenance of the equilibrium across the cell membrane, and when the calcium ion concentration is low, the excitability of the nerve is increased.

When a stimulus is applied to an axon, the selective permeability of the cell membrane is altered, which allows an inrush of sodium ions into the cell. This causes a reduction of the resting potential difference across the membrane. If the membrane potential is lowered (depolarized) to a critical level (30–50 mV), an *action potential* results and the impulse is propagated along the cell membrane as a wave of depolarization. In non-myelinated fibres there is a continuous flow of the impulse as ionic eddies excite the neighbouring membrane. The rate of spread of the impulse is proportional to the cross-sectional area of the axon.

Conduction of the impulse in myelinated fibres occurs in a saltatory manner; the impulse or wave of membrane depolarization skips from one node of Ranvier to the next. Myelin acts as an insulator and prevents excitation of the axon cell membrane except where there are gaps in the sheath at the node of Ranvier. Increased permeability of the excited membrane at the node to sodium ions causes ionic currents to flow to the next node and the current to flow in the reverse direction in the endoneurial fluid. When the current density reaches the threshold level, depolarization initiates similar permeability changes at the next node of Ranvier. As the flow of ions through the cytoplasm is much more rapid than the spread of the wave of depolarization along the cell membrane, higher conduction velocities are reached by saltatory conduction. Some radial leak of current occurs through the membrane sheath, and from theoretical considerations Rushton (1951) predicted that the optimal ratio (g) of an axon diameter to total fibre diameter (i.e. axon plus myelin) for saltatory conduction would be 0·6, but, as Williams and Wendell-Smith (1971) have shown, this optimal ratio is attained only in the larger myelinated fibres. In addition to axon diameter and myelin sheath thickness, the distance between nodes (internodal length) is important in determining the speed of conduction. This varies from 200 μm to more than 1000 μm in larger fibres; thus the ratio of internodal length to axon diameter may be 100:1.

Most peripheral nerve fascicles have a mixed population of nerve fibres which vary in diameter; some are myelinated but many are non-myelinated. After synchronous stimulation, conduction along nerve trunks results in a Compound Action Potential which is the summation of different conduction velocities. Four main peaks are seen in a compound action potential, viz. α, β, γ and δ, representing groups of fibres conducting at different velocities. Clinically, conduction velocities of nerve trunks are measured through the skin and vary in value from 58–72 m s^{-1} in the radial nerve to 47–51 m s^{-1} in the peroneal nerve (Smorto and Basmajian, 1972).

MYELINATED NERVE FIBRES

Many of the early investigators of peripheral nerve structure recognized the value of examining lengths of individually teased myelinated fibres in addition to cross-sections of nerve. A myelinated nerve fibre is divided into segments, each representing the length of a single Schwann cell and the myelin sheath which that cell has produced. The axon is continuous from segment to segment, whereas nodes of Ranvier mark the junction between segments and the small gap between consecutive Schwann cells. The distance between each node of Ranvier is the internodal length and, in a normal nerve, it is proportional to the total diameter (axon plus myelin sheath) of the fibre. The nucleus of the Schwann cell (*Figure 14*) is usually situated near the mid-point of the internode. Internodal lengths are determined by the amount of growth of the nerve that occurs after myelination has commenced. When myelination begins in embryonic life or early childhood, the Schwann cells are spaced along the nerve; each cell length is approximately 300 µm, which is the average length of Schwann cell in tissue culture. As the body grows and with it the length of the nerve, the number of Schwann cells along a myelinated fibre remains constant and the internodal length increases with the growth of the body. The larger-diameter axons start myelinating earlier in development than the smaller axons and this correlates well with the observation that larger-

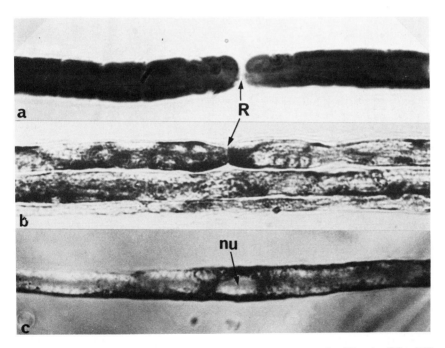

Fig. 14. Teased myelinated nerve fibres: (a) Stained with osmium; node of Ranvier (R). × 700 (b) NADH-tetrazolium reductase technique showing staining of cytoplasm around the node of Ranvier (R). × 760 (Courtesy of Brain.) (c) Internodal portion of a fibre stained by NADH-tetrazolium reductase technique. The nucleus (nu) is outlined by stained cytoplasm. × 760 (Courtesy of Brain)

diameter myelinated fibres have the longer internodes, e.g. a 2 µm diameter axon has an internodal length of approximately 0·15 mm and in a 12 µm diameter fibre the internodal length is 1–1·2 µm (Lascelles and Thomas, 1966). Following segmental demyelination or axonal degeneration in an adult nerve, the original long internode may be remyelinated by several Schwann cells, each with the embryonic internodal length of 300 µm (Fullerton *et al.*, 1965).

The thickness of the myelin sheath measured in transverse sections of normal peripheral nerve is proportional to the diameter of the axon. This feature is very useful for detecting axons that are remyelinating following segmental demyelination, for in this situation axons with disproportionately thin myelin sheaths are observed (see Chapter 4).

In a large proportion of its internodal length the myelinated fibre is roughly circular in cross-section. However, there is distortion of the contour in the nuclear region but more especially at the node of Ranvier and in the adjacent paranodal region. *Figures 10* and *17* show that myelinated fibres are elliptical in cross-section in the nuclear regions. Williams and Landon (1963) emphasized the changes in shape of myelinated fibres in the paranodal region, particularly in large-diameter fibres. The myelin sheath is fluted and the surface groove filled with cytoplasm rich in mitochondria (*Figure 14b*), which probably reflects the high metabolic requirements of the region. In addition to the fluting, which is best seen in transverse sections, the paranodal region is seen to be slightly bulbous in teased fibres. The cytoplasm in the grooves of the fluted myelin sheaths can be seen in teased preparation stained for mitochondrial enzymes. Other irregularities in the myelin sheaths are often seen in the paranodal region, usually in the form of loops or tongues of myelin extending from the sheath (Webster and Spiro, 1960).

ULTRASTRUCTURE OF MYELINATED NERVE FIBRES

The axon

Axons of myelinated fibres vary in diameter from small 3 µm diameter fibres to the large axons of 15–20 µm diameter fibres. They can be demonstrated with a light microscope by various silver techniques and histochemically by mitochondrial stains. In 1 µm toluidine blue stained Araldite sections (*Figure 10*), normal axons are virtually unstained. Electron microscopy reveals a limiting plasma membrane (axolemma) around the axon which is separated from the enveloping Schwann cell membrane by a gap approximately 20 nm wide. Within the cytoplasm there are long, thin mitochondria orientated along the long axis and seen in cross-section as small, round profiles, usually of 150–300 nm diameter. A number of single membrane-bound elongated profiles are present and probably represent fragments of a continuous smooth endoplasmic reticular network (*Figure 15*). Multivesicular bodies are also found in the axoplasm. The most prominent components of the axon are the neurofilaments and neurotubules (*Figure 15*). In the larger axons the 10 nm diameter neurofilaments are the more numerous and are most densely packed at the node of Ranvier, where there is slight narrowing of the axon. The tubules are 20 nm in diameter and have an

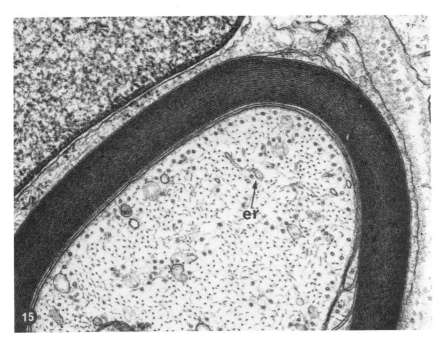

Fig. 15. Electron micrograph of a peripheral nerve fibre cut in transverse section. The axon contains many neurofilaments appearing as dots in the transverse section; the neurotubules are more prominent at the periphery. Smooth endoplasmic reticulum (er). × 37 500

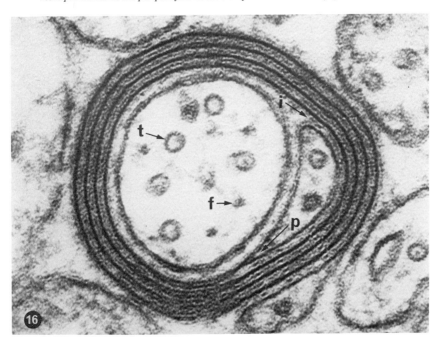

Fig. 16. Electron micrograph of a small myelinated fibre in a rabbit brain. Neurotubules (t) and neurofilaments (f) are seen in the axon. Formation of myelin period line (p) and interperiod line (i) from oligodendrocyte cell membrane is also shown. × 220 000

45

unstained central 'lumen' (*Figure 15*). They are composed of pairs of globular sub-units of 4·5 nm diameter arranged in a spiral so that in transverse section the circumference of the tubule presents 13 such units (*Figure 16*). This arrangement suggests that tubules are formed by spirals of dimer sub-units and may be polymerized neurofibrils (Erickson, 1974). Delicate processes or side arms can often be seen radiating from filaments and microtubules. The basic structure of neurotubules is similar to microtubules in other cells and seen especially in cilia and mitotic spindles. Colchicine and various antimitotic agents, especially vinca alkaloids, bind to neurotubular protein and prevent the formation of neurotubules.

Axoplasmic transport

The metabolic dependence of the axon upon the neurone soma is illustrated when the distal portion of the transected axon degenerates (Waller, 1850). This suggests in itself that there is some flow of cell components from the neuronal perikaryon along the axon to its distal end. Weiss and Hiscoe (1948), however, showed also that when an axon is constricted, cytoplasm and cell organelles accumulate proximal to the constriction.

With the introduction of isotopes and other labelling techniques it became clear that there are different rates of neuronofugal axoplasmic transport. Cell organelles such as mitochondria, lysosomes and vesicles move at a *slow rate* of $1-3$ mm day^{-1} (Lasek, 1967), whereas selected proteins and other material move at the fast rate of 100 mm day^{-1} (Ochs, 1972). Catecholamine storage granules in sympathetic nerves are transported at varying speeds of $2-10$ mm h^{-1} ($48-240$ mm day^{-1}), depending upon the species (Dahlström, 1967), and neurosecretory granules in the hypothalamo–hypophyseal tract move at 2800 mm day^{-1}.

The exact mechanism of axoplasmic transport is not known, but neurotubules and neurofilaments are thought to be in some way connected with the fast component of axoplasmic flow. Evidence for this hypothesis stems from the observation that colchicine not only interferes with rapid axoplasmic transport (Ochs, 1972), but also binds to microtubular protein sub-units (Borisy and Taylor, 1967) and prevents the formation of microtubules (Wisniewski, Terry and Hirano, 1970). Droz *et al.* (1974) have recently proposed that rapid axoplasmic transport is associated with the extensive membranous reticular system which extends from the neurone cell body into the axon.

Much emphasis has been placed upon axoplasmic flow along the axon away from the neurone cell body, but there is now substantial evidence for retrograde axoplasmic transport of material from nerve terminal to neuronal cell body (Kristensson and Olsson, 1973). A marker protein, horse-radish peroxidase, injected into the tongue of a rat or rabbit will be taken up by the distal ends of the motor fibres and transported to the cell bodies of the hypoglossal neurones at 120 mm day^{-1}. This mechanism not only has physiological implications, but is also of pathological importance, particularly as viruses such as herpes simplex are transported in this way (Blinzinger and Anzil, 1974). Botulinum and tetanus toxins enter nerve endings and may be carried to the neuronal soma by retrograde transport (Kristensson and Olssen, 1973). The mechanism of retrograde transport is not known.

Schwann cell and myelin sheath

Schwann cells normally have a closely investing layer of basement membrane (*Figure 17*) which distinguishes them from endoneurial fibroblasts. The continuity of the basement membrane tube across the node of Ranvier from segment to segment is thought to play an important role in establishing a 'Schwann tube' pathway for regenerating axons after nerve section. Most of the Schwann cytoplasm in the larger myelinated fibres is concentrated around the node of Ranvier and in the perinuclear region (*Figure 14*). The nucleus lies outside the myelin sheath and the perinuclear cytoplasm contains smooth-surfaced endoplasmic reticulum, Golgi cisterns, mitochondria and polyribosomes (*Figure 17*); very little rough-surfaced endoplasmic reticulum is seen in normal unreactive Schwann cells. In histochemical preparations of older human nerves there is intense acid phosphatase staining in the perinuclear region; this enzyme activity is associated with the π-granules of Reich (1903) (Noback, 1953), which stain metachromatically with toluidine blue in frozen sections; π-granules cannot be so stained in paraffin sections. Ultrastructurally, π-granules consist of lamellated structures and amorphous osmiophilic globules (Weller and Herzog, 1970; Tomonaga and Sluga, 1970) and they are probably analogous to lipofuschin seen in other long-lived cells. Very few π-granules are seen in the nerves of patients with chronic peripheral neuropathies where there has been extensive Schwann cell mitosis and replication (Weller and Herzog, 1970).

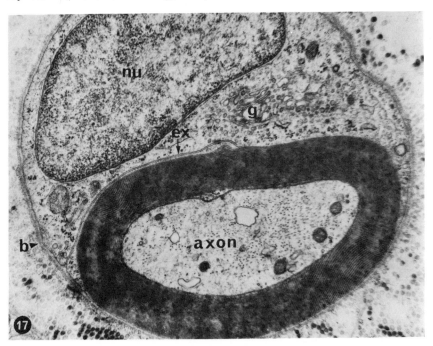

Fig. 17. T.S. human myelinated nerve fibre through the nuclear region. Nucleus (nu), Golgi apparatus (g), basement membranes (b), external mesaxon (ex). Electron micrograph × 19 520 (Courtesy of J. Neurol. Neurosurg. Psychiat.)

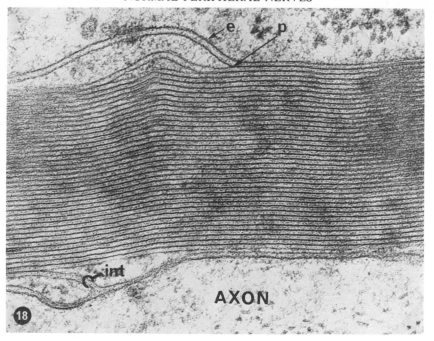

Fig. 18. Peripheral nerve myelin. The cytoplasmic aspects of the cell membrane fuse to form the dense period line (p) at the external mesaxon (e); the interperiod line is indistinct. Internal mesaxon (int). × 117 000 (Courtesy of J. Neurol. Neurosurg. Psychiat.*)*

Myelin is formed by the fusion of layers of Schwann cell membrane (*Figure 18*; Geren, 1954) forming a tight spiral wrapping around the axon. During fetal development Schwann cells insinuate themselves into groups of naked axons and partition off smaller and smaller groups (Cravioto, 1965; Davison and Peters, 1970). Finally, certain Schwann cells enclose only one axon, usually the larger-diameter axons, and these are destined to become myelinated. The axon lies at first in a furrow on the surface of the Schwann cell but later becomes invaginated into the cell, and the lips of the furrow become closely opposed, to form the mesaxon. At this stage the future myelinated axon is in a similar position to a mature non-myelinated axon. Following invagination, tongues of Schwann cytoplasm extend around the axon in a spiral; the cytoplasm is expelled from the spiral as the layers of Schwann cell membrane become compacted to form myelin (Geren, 1954). Often the outer layers of the sheath are compacted first, leaving a rim of cytoplasm on the inner aspect of the myelin sheath which finally disappears as the fibre matures. The original connection with the Schwann cell surface is still maintained as the external mesaxon; its counterpart on the inner aspect of the myelin sheath is the internal mesaxon, where the Schwann cell membranes separate to enclose the axon (*Figure 18*). A periaxonal space of 20 nm between the axon plasma membrane and the inner Schwann cell membrane is maintained for most of the internode, but specialized junctional areas may be seen at the node of Ranvier (*Figure 22*). A roughly analogous situation exists in the central nervous system, where the myelin sheath is formed from compacted oligodendroglial cell membrane (*Figure 16*). Each oligodendroglial cell myelinates several axons (Bunge, 1968); a separate cell process extends to wrap around each axon. Nodes of Ranvier are very similar in structure to those in the peripheral nervous system and the transition of central to peripheral myelin sheath takes place at nodes of Ranvier in the nerve root entry zone in the spinal cord or brain stem.

In osmium-fixed tissue the cell membrane is a trilaminar structure 7·0–7·5 nm in thickness, composed of two outer stained bands 2–2·5 nm thick, separated by a pale zone. The inner, cytoplasmic aspect of the membrane is a densely staining continuous black line, whereas the outer aspect of the membrane is less distinct. During the formation of the myelin sheath the cytoplasmic aspects of the Schwann cell membranes fuse to form a densely osmiophilic 'period line' and the outer aspects of the membrane fuse to form a less distinct 'interperiod line' (*Figure 18*).

X-ray diffraction studies of myelin reveal a periodicity (i.e. distance between two period lines) of 17·0–18·0 nm (Finean, 1953, 1965). From these measurements various molecular models have been constructed (Finean, 1953, 1965; Vandenheuvel, 1968). These suggest that the myelin lipids, cholesterol, cerebroside and phospholipid form a bimolecular leaflet 5·0 nm thick, which occupies the unstained region in the electron micrographs. The major part of the protein is thought to be situated in the stained regions of the myelin (i.e. period and interperiod lines) (Benson, 1966; Davison and Peters, 1970).

Owing to shrinkage and the extraction of lipids during preparation, the myelin sheath in electron micrographs has a periodicity of approximately 12·0 nm. The distinct period line is usually single but the interperiod line may be split, and this gap is apparently still in continuity with the extracellular space (Revel and Hamilton, 1969).

Schmidt–Lanterman incisures

Funnel-shaped discontinuities in the myelin sheath are seen along the myelinated fibres (*Figure 19*). These are Schmidt–Lantermann incisures and were thought for many years to be artefact. Recent studies, however, have shown that although they are often greatly exaggerated in paraffin sections, they do have a real anatomical basis. Hall and Williams (1970) observed dilatation of the incisures in *in vivo* preparations of mouse nerve when hypotonic solutions were applied, and, conversely, the incisures closed under hypertonic conditions. Ultrastructurally, the period line of the myelin sheath in the region of the incisure splits to enclose Schwann cytoplasm including microtubules and vesicles (*Figure 20*); the interperiod line may also separate. Stacks of desmosomoid structures are seen within the incisure, especially in the outer portion of the myelin sheath (Hall and Williams, 1970). The incisures are, in effect, tracts of Schwann cytoplasm spiralling through the myelin sheath. It has been suggested that they may be pathways of intracellular transport of metabolites concerned with the economy of either the Schwann cell or the axon. Alternatively, the incisures may be related to myelinated fibre growth and remodelling.

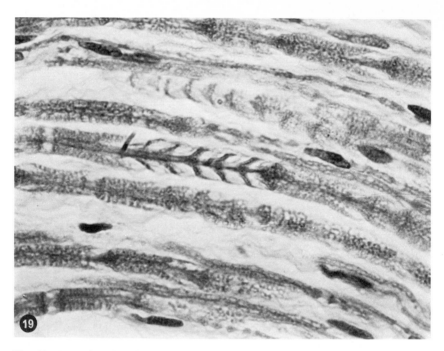

Fig. 19. Arrow-shaped Schmidt–Lantermann incisures in an L.S. paraffin section of nerve stained with H. and E. × 788

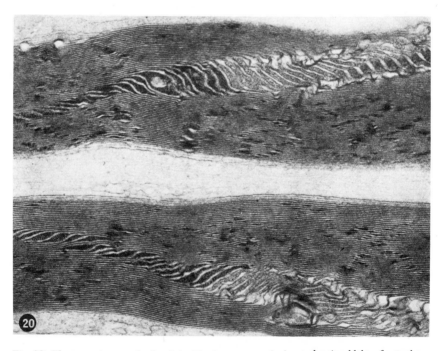

Fig. 20. Electron micrograph of a Schmidt–Lantermann incisure showing blebs of cytoplasm between separated myelin lamellae. × 40 000

50

Node of Ranvier

The ultrastructure of the node of Ranvier and the paranodal region is rather more complex in the larger myelinated fibres than in the small-diameter fibres. Not only is it the region where consecutive Schwann cells meet and the internodal myelin sheath ends, but it is also an important functional area of ion exchange between extracellular fluid and the axon during saltatory conduction of the nerve impulse.

In smaller fibres the few lamellae in the relatively thin myelin sheath terminate at an acute angle at the node as a regular series of end-loops containing cytoplasm, microtubules and ribosomes (*Figures 21* and *22*). There are often stacks of desmosomoid structures between the end-loops. Periodic densities may be seen in the gap between the Schwann cell membrane of the end-loop and the axon plasma membrane (Bunge *et al.*, 1967).

Tongues of Schwann cytoplasm extend beyond the termination of the myelin sheath and interdigitate with the adjacent Schwann cell forming the other half of the node (*Figure 21*). Thus, there is little bare axon surface devoid of Schwann cell covering. The 'nodal gap', i.e. the gap between consecutive segments of myelin sheath, is well demonstrated in teased fibres; it is for the most part filled with cytoplasm.

In large-diameter fibres the myelin sheath in the paranodal region either side of the node of Ranvier is crenated in cross-section and the grooves are filled with tongues of cytoplasm radiating from the nodal region. These tongues are

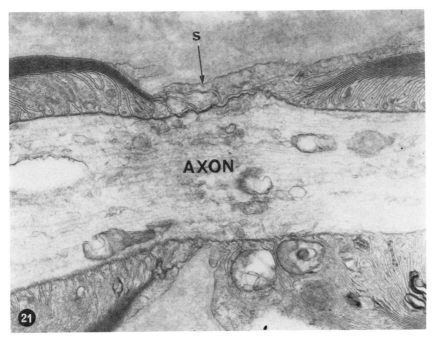

Fig. 21. A node of Ranvier showing the myelin end-loops and Schwann cell processes (s) closely applied to the axon. Electron micrograph × 24 700

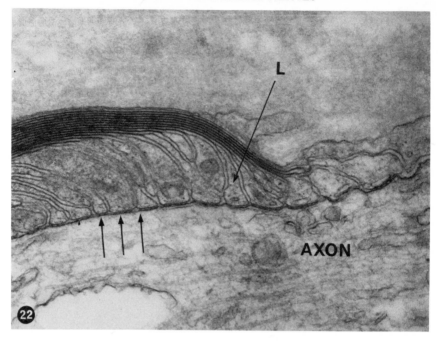

Fig. 22. Higher-power view of myelin loops (L) at a node of Ranvier. There are focal densities between the loop membrane and the axon plasma membrane (arrows). Electron micrograph × 47 700

rich in mitochondria and probably reflect high metabolic activity at the node (Williams and Landon, 1963). In addition to the fluting of the paranodal region, irregular tongues of myelin project from the sheath and form a complicated pattern (Webster and Spiro, 1960). It is important to recognize this feature, as it may be mistaken for a pathological feature in nerve biopsies.

The pattern formed at the node by the terminal end-loops in large fibres may be very complex. Furthermore, the myelin lamellae in the thicker sheaths are almost perpendicular to the axon at the node, which produces a rounded profile of the sheath at the node. Within the gap between the consecutive myelin sheaths there is a complex array of delicate finger-like Schwann cell processes which converge upon the axon like a spiny bracelet (Landon and Williams, 1963). These processes are embedded in a circular collar of sulphated mucopolysaccharide (glucosaminoglucuronoglycans) (Langley and Landon, 1968) which binds various cations (Langley, 1969) and might well play an important part in ion exchange at the node of Ranvier. Histochemical preparations also suggest that acetylcholine esterase is present in the nodal gap region (Adams, Bayliss and Grant, 1968).

NON-MYELINATED NERVE FIBRES

The majority of axons in a normal mixed peripheral nerve are small, non-myelinated fibres less than 3 μm in diameter (Ochoa and Mair, 1969a). Several

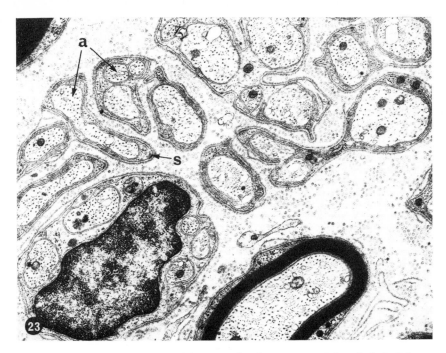

Fig. 23. T.S. non-myelinated axons (a) in an infant human nerve. Relatively little Schwann cytoplasm (s) is associated with each axon. Electron micrograph × 9900 (Courtesy of J. Neurol. Neurosurg. Psychiat.)

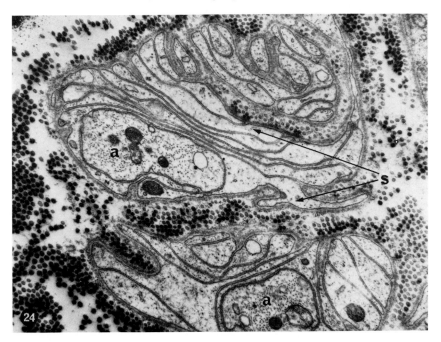

Fig. 24. Non-myelinated axons (a) in an adult human nerve showing the associated stacks of Schwann cell processes (s). Electron micrograph × 18 000

non-myelinated axons are invaginated into a single Schwann cell or its processes and connected to the surface by a mesaxon (*Figure 23*). The axons contain microtubules, neurofilaments, mitochondria and vesicles. A gap of 20 nm separates the axon cell membrane from the enveloping Schwann cell; acetyl cholinesterase activity can be detected within this gap (Pearse, 1972).

The Schwann cells are arranged in series along the groups of non-myelinated axons and the terminal processes of consecutive Schwann cells interdigitate with each other (Eames and Gamble, 1970) but with no obvious area that corresponds to the node of Ranvier in the myelinated fibre. This arrangement reflects the different modes of neural conduction, i.e. continuous propagation of the impulse along the non-myelinated axon and saltatory conduction in the myelinated fibre.

Axon–Schwann cell relationships are relatively simple in young human subjects and very similar in arrangement to those observed in laboratory mammals (*Figure 23*; Weller, 1967). In older people, however, the Schwann cell processes proliferate and form tightly packed stacks (*Figure 24*; Weller, 1967; Ochoa and Mair, 1969b). This may reflect progressive damage and fibre degeneration in older nerves, possibly with gradual depletion of non-myelinated axons.

NERVE ENDINGS

Neural transmission between one neuron and another takes place across the synapse. In the central nervous system axons terminate as bulbous presynaptic 'boutons terminaux' which form synapses on the surface of the neurone cell body or a dendrite. Each presynaptic bouton contains synaptic vesicles carrying neural transmitter substance. Vesicles containing acetyl choline are electron-lucid, whereas vesicles containing catecholamines have a dense osmiophilic core, and are not only seen in the terminal boutons, but can also be traced electron microscopically and by formalin fluorescence (Dahlström, 1967) along the axons.

The cell membranes on either side of the synaptic gap show specialized dense areas. Synaptic transmission occurs when the impulse arrives at the bouton and transmitter substance is released following fusion of the synaptic vesicles with the presynaptic membrane. The postsynaptic membrane is depolarized and the transmitter substance is either hydrolysed by acetylcholine esterase (cholinergic endings) or may be largely taken up again by the terminal bouton (as occurs with catecholamines).

Transmitter substances are released from peripheral nerve endings outside the central nervous system or ganglia in a way that is basically very similar to their release in the central nervous system. There are two main types of peripheral release site, i.e. simple endings of autonomic nerves on smooth muscle or secretory cells and the rather more complex myoneural junctions where motor nerves terminate in relation to muscle end-plates.

MUSCLE END-PLATES

Nerves supplying somatic extrafusal muscle fibres branch within the muscle and innervate varying numbers of muscle fibres, from a few to many hundreds, depending upon the muscle. The innervation zone is usually concentrated in the central region of the muscle. This zone can be localized in the muscle by electrical stimulation and demonstrated histologically by staining the muscle end-plates for cholinesterase. The nerve endings are seen in silver-stained preparations (Schofield technique) and are well demonstrated by intravital staining with methylene blue (Coërs, 1952). Just proximal to the myoneural junction, the nerve branch loses its myelin sheath and breaks up into a terminal arborization of unmyelinated twigs; each nerve terminal contains synaptic vesicles and lies within a trough in the surface of the muscle end-plate. The ultrastructure of the neuromuscular junction in man is similar to that in other mammals. There is, however, some structural difference between the end-plates of slow (Type 1), fast (Type 2) and intermediate muscle fibres (Padykula and Gauthier, 1970).

The end-plate is near the mid-point of the muscle fibre and is devoid of myofibrils. It is seen as a depression in the surface of the fibre with parallel gutters in the floor of the trough. An unmyelinated terminal lies in each of the synaptic troughs partly covered by Schwann cell processes. A layer of basement membrane separates the bulbous terminal axon from the muscle end-plate surface. Synaptic vesicles within the terminal axon contain acetyl choline; cholinesterase is localized to the gap between the nerve terminal and the end-plate. Depolarization of the muscle end-plate occurs following release of acetyl choline from the synaptic vesicles, and the propagation of an action potential is initiated in the muscle fibre (Zaimis and MacLagan, 1974). In large muscle fibres the action potential is thought to be conducted throughout the depths of the fibre along a special tubular system. Electrical stimulation spread in this way causes the release of calcium from the sarcoplasmic reticulum deep within the muscle fibre and results in activation of the contractile elements (actin and myosin) in the immediate vicinity.

SENSORY RECEPTORS

Apart from the special sensory organs such as the eye, ear, vestibular apparatus, olfactory organ and taste buds, there are many types of sensory receptors which vary in function and structural complexity. Visceral (interoceptive) sensation is mainly mediated by the simple nerve endings on blood vessels and those distributed throughout various organs. Somatic sensation may be divided into exteroceptive and proprioceptive.

Exteroceptive sensibility is concerned with the appreciation of stimuli from outside the body and includes the special sense organs and cutaneous sensation. Various classifications of cutaneous end-organs exist, and they are based mainly upon structural characteristics but to some extent upon function (Warwick and Williams, 1973).

(a) *Free nerve endings* are present in the skin related to hair follicles or enveloped by epithelial cells as in the cornea. They are small myelinated and non-myelinated fibres (group III) mainly concerned with pain and itch.

(b) *Corpuscular endings.* Several different types of ending have been described. (i) Meissner's tactile corpuscles in the papillae of the skin are approximately 80×30 μm and composed of lamellar cells. They are associated with the sensation of fine touch. (ii) Pacinian corpuscles are composed of up to

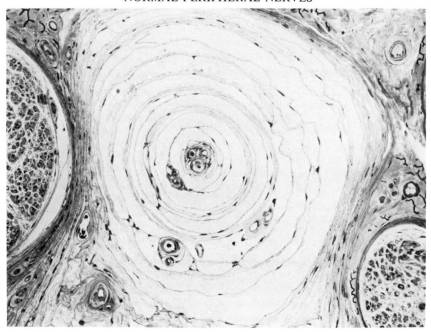

Fig. 25. Pacinian corpuscle in a sural nerve showing a central core surrounded by multiple widely spaced cellular lamellae. 1 μm Araldite section stained with toluidine blue. × 158

30 concentric lamellae forming a corpuscle 100–500 μm in diameter (Spencer and Schaumberg, 1973). They are situated in subcutaneous tissue, mesentery, pancreas and a variety of other sites, including the epineurium of peripheral nerve (*Figure 25*). They are rapidly adapting receptors which respond to local light pressure (Boyd and Davey, 1968). Various other histological varieties of corpuscular endings are recognized, e.g. bulbous corpuscles of Krause (Warwick and Williams, 1973).

Proprioceptive sensations are concerned with the appreciation of the posture and movement of the body itself; they are derived from the labyrinths, muscles, tendons and joints. The sensory endings around the joints have a range of structure (Warwick and Williams, 1973). Within the limb muscles there are bare sensory nerve endings and Golgi tendon organs, but the most complex of the muscle sensory organs is the muscle spindle.

Muscle spindles

Muscle spindles are distributed throughout skeletal muscles. They are sensory receptors that respond to stretch of the muscle and relay information about the length and rate of change of length in the extrafusal muscle fibres. Sensory nerve impulses from muscle spindles initiate the stretch reflex and provide a feed-back mechanism which controls the force of muscle contraction (Matthews, 1964, 1972).

Each spindle is several millimetres long and consists of a number of intrafusal muscle fibres surrounded by a loose capsule; their structure is very similar in most mammalian species that have been examined (Price, 1974). There are two types of intrafusal muscle fibre. One type, the nuclear-chain fibres, do not usually run the whole length of the muscle spindle; they are 7–20 μm in diameter and there are usually 3–7 per spindle. Each fibre has a chain-like arrangement of nuclei in the central sensory region; the polar ends of the fibres contain striated muscle fibrils and have a motor innervation. The other type, the nuclear-bag intrafusal fibres, have 40–50 nuclei clumped together near the equator of the fibre, which is also the sensory region. There are one or two nuclear-bag fibres running the whole length of the muscle spindle. The polar ends of these fibres also contain striated contractile elements which are innervated by small myelinated fibres arising from small neurones in the anterior horns of the spinal cord.

The sensory endings on muscle spindles have been extensively studied (Boyd, 1962; Swash and Fox, 1972), and there are several accounts of their ultrastructure (see Scalzi and Price, 1971). Impulses from primary sensory annulospiral nerve endings around the central regions of nuclear-chain and nuclear-bag fibres are conducted by large myelinated fibres. The response is excitation of motor neurones supplying synergistic muscles and inhibition of neurones innervating antagonistic muscles. Secondary sensory annulospiral endings are around nuclear-chain intrafusal fibres and the impulses travel in slowly conducting small nerve fibres to influence motor neurones through inter-neurones in the spinal cord.

Functionally, the primary and secondary annulospiral sensory endings are sensitive to stretch (Matthews, 1964, 1972). The nuclear-bag fibres are concerned with position and velocity sense (dynamic response), whereas the nuclear-chain fibres adapt more slowly and are concerned with the static response. Through the motor supply to the polar contractile regions the length of both types of intrafusal fibre can be adjusted to compensate for changes in length of the extrafusal muscle fibres.

REFERENCES

Adams, C. W. M., Bayliss, O. B. and Grant, R. T. (1968). 'Cholinesterases in peripheral nervous system. III. Validity of localisation around the node of Ranvier.' *Histochem. J.*, **1**, 68.

Adams, W. E. (1943). 'The blood supply of nerves. II. The effects of the exclusion of its regional sources of supply on the sciatic nerve of the rabbit.' *J. Anat.*, **77**, 243.

Aguayo, A. J., Martin, J. B. and Bray, G. M. (1972). 'Effects of nerve growth factor antiserum on peripheral unmyelinated nerve fibres.' *Acta Neuropath. (Berlin)*, **20**, 288.

Andrew, A. (1971). 'The origin of intramural ganglia. IV. The origin of enteric ganglia: a critical review and discussion of the present state of the problem.' *J. Anat.*, **108**, 169.

Asbury, A. K. (1973). 'Renaut bodies: a forgotten endoneurial structure.' *J. Neuropath. Exp. Neurol.*, **32**, 334–343.

Benson, A. A. (1966). 'On the orientation of lipid in chloroplast and cell membranes.' *J. Am. Oil Chem. Soc.*, **43**, 265.

Blinzinger, K. and Anzil, A. P. (1974). 'Neural route of infection in virus diseases of the central nervous system.' *Lancet*, **ii,** 1374.

Borisy, G. G. and Taylor, E. W. (1967). 'The mechanism of action of colchicine. Colchicine binding to sea urchin eggs and the mitotic apparatus.' *J. Cell Biol.*, **34**, 535.

Boyd, I. A. (1962). 'The structure and innervation of the nuclear bag muscle fibre system and the nuclear chain muscle fibre system in mammalian muscle spindles.' *Phil. Trans. B*, **245**, 81.

REFERENCES

Boyd, I. A. and Davey, M. R. (1968). In *Composition of Peripheral Nerves*. Edinburgh; Livingstone.

Brain, W. R. and Walton, J. N. (1969). In *Brain's Diseases of the Nervous System*, 7th edn. London; Oxford University Press.

Brodal, A. (1969). In *Neurological Anatomy in Relation to Clinical Medicine*, 2nd edn. London; Oxford University Press.

Bunge, M. B., Bunge, R.P., Peterson, E. R. and Murray, M. R. (1967). 'A light and electron microscope study of long-term organised cultures of rat dorsal root ganglia.' *J. Cell Biol.*, **32**, 439.

Bunge, R. P. (1968). 'Glial cells and the central myelin sheath.' *Physiol. Rev.*, **48**, 197.

Coërs, C. (1952). 'The vital staining of muscle biopsies with methylene blue.' *J. Neurol. Neurosurg. Psychiat.*, **15**, 211.

Cravioto, H. (1965). 'The rôle of Schwann cells in the development of human peripheral nerves. An electron microscope study.' *J. Ultrastruct. Res.*, **12**, 634.

Dahlström, A. (1967). 'Transport of catecholamine storage granules.' In *Axoplasmic Transport*. Ed. by S. H. Barondes. *Neurosciences Research Program Bulletin*, **5**, 317.

Davison, A. N. and Peters, A. (1970). In *Myelination*. Springfield, Illinois; Charles C. Thomas.

Droz, B., Bennett, G., di Giamberardino, L., Koenig, H. L. and Rambourg, A. (1974). 'Contribution of electron microscopy to the study of axonal flow.' In *Proc. VIIth International Congress of Neuropathology, Budapest, 1974*.

Dyck, P. J. and Hopkins, A. P. (1972). 'Electron microscopic observations on degeneration and regeneration of unmyelinated fibres.' *Brain*, **95**, 223.

Eames, R. A. and Gamble, H. J. (1970). 'Schwann cell relationships in normal human cutaneous nerves.' *J. Anat.*, **106**, 417.

Erickson, H. P. (1974). 'Microtubule surface lattice and sub-unit structure and observations on reassembly.' *J. Cell. Biol.*, **60**, 153.

Farquhar, M. G. and Palade, G. E. (1963). 'Junctional complexes in various epithelia.' *J. Cell Biol.*, **17**, 375.

Finean, J. B. (1953). 'Phospholipid–cholesterol complex in structure of myelin.' *Experimentia*, **9**, 17.

Finean, J. B. (1965). 'Molecular parameters in the nerve myelin sheath.' *Ann. N.Y. Acad. Sci.*, **122**, 51.

Fraher, J. P. (1972). 'A quantitative study of anterior root fibres during early myelination.' *J. Anat.*, **112**, 99.

Fullerton, P. M., Gilliatt, R. W., Lascelles, R. G. and Morgan-Hughes, J. A. (1965). 'Relation between fibre diameter and internodal length in chronic neuropathy.' *J. Physiol. (London)*, **178**, 26P.

Gamble, H. J. and Eames, R. A. (1964). 'An electron microscopic study of the connective tissues of human peripheral nerve.' *J. Anat.*, **98**, 655.

Gamble, H. G. and Eames, R. A. (1966). 'Electron microscopy of human spinal nerve roots.' *Arch. Neurol.*, **14**, 50.

Geren, B. B. (1954). 'The formation from the Schwann cell surface of myelin in the peripheral nerves of chick embryos.' *Exp. Cell Res.*, **7**, 558.

Hall, S. M. and Williams, P. L. (1970). 'Studies on the "incisures" of Schmidt and Lanterman.' *J. Cell Sci.*, **6**, 767.

King, R. H. M. and Thomas, P. K. (1971). 'Electron microscope observations on aberrant regeneration of unmyelinated axons in the vagus nerve of the rabbit.' *Acta Neuropath. (Berlin)*, **18**, 150.

Kristensson, K. and Olsson, Y. (1973). 'Diffusion, pathways and retrograde axonal transport of protein tracers in peripheral nerves.' *Progr. Neurobiol.*, **1**, 85.

Landon, D. N. and Williams, P. L. (1963). 'Ultrastructure of the node of Ranvier.' *Nature (London)*, **199**, 575.

Langley, O. K. (1969). 'Ion-exchange at the node of Ranvier.' *Histochem. J.*, **1**, 295.

Langley, O. K. and Landon, D. N. (1968). 'A light and electron histochemical approach to the node of Ranvier and the myelin of peripheral nerve fibres.' *J. Histochem. Cytochem.*, **15**, 722.

Lascelles, R. G. and Thomas, P. K. (1966). 'Changes due to age in internodal length in the sural nerve of man.' *J. Neurol. Neurosurg. Psychiat.*, **29**, 40.

Lasek, R. J. (1967). 'Slow and rapid transport of proteins.' In *Axoplasmic Transport*. Ed. by S. H. Barondes. *Neurosciences Research Program Bulletin*, **5**, 314.

Levi-Montalcini, R. and Angeletti, P. U. (1968). 'Nerve growth factor.' *Physiol. Rev.*, **48**, 534.

Matthews, P. B. C. (1964). 'Muscle spindles and their motor control.' *Physiol. Rev.*, **44**, 219.

REFERENCES

Matthews, P. B. C. (1972). *Mammalian Muscle Receptors and their Central Actions*. London; Edward Arnold.

Noback, C. R. (1953). 'The protagon (π) granules of Reich.' *J. Comp. Neurol.*, **99**, 91.

Ochoa, J. and Mair, W. G. P. (1969a). 'The normal sural nerve in man. I. Ultrastructure and numbers of fibres and cells.' *Acta Neuropath. (Berlin)*, **13**, 197.

Ochoa, J. and Mair, W. G. P. (1969b). 'The normal sural nerve in man. II. Changes in the axons and Schwann cells due to ageing.' *Acta Neuropath. (Berlin)*, **13**, 217.

Ochs, S. (1972). 'Fast transport of materials in mammalian nerve fibres.' *Science, N.Y.*, **176**, 252.

Olsson, Y. (1968). 'Studies on vascular permeability in peripheral nerves. 3. Permeability changes in vasa nervorum and exudation of serum albumin in INH-induced neuropathy in the rat.' *Acta Neuropath. (Berlin)*, **11**, 103.

Olsson, Y. (1971). 'Mast cells in human peripheral nerve.' *Acta Neurol. Scand.*, **47**, 357.

Padykula, H. A. and Gauthier, G. F. (1970). 'The ultrastructure of the neuromuscular junctions of mammalian red, white and intermediate skeletal muscle fibres.' *J. Cell Biol.*, **46**, 27.

Paintal, A. S. (1973). *Conduction in Mammalian Nerve Fibres. New Developments in Electromyography and Clinical Neurophysiology*, Vol. 2, pp. 19–41. Ed. by J. E. Desmedt. Basle; Karger.

Pearse, A. G. E. (1972). In *Histochemistry—Theoretical and Applied*, 3rd edn, Vol. 2. Edinburgh; Churchill Livingstone.

Price, H. M. (1974). 'Ultrastructure of the skeletal muscle fibre.' In *Disorders of Voluntary Muscle*, 3rd edn. Ed. by J. N. Walton. Edinburgh; Churchill Livingstone.

Reich, F. (1903). 'Über eine neue Granulation in der Nervenzelle.' *Arch. Anat. Physiol., Physiol. Abt.*, 208.

Revel, J.-P. and Hamilton, D. W. (1969). 'The double nature of the intermediate dense line in peripheral nerve myelin.' *Anat. Rec.*, **163**, 7.

Rushton, W. A. H. (1951). 'A theory of the effects of fibre size in medullated nerve.' *J. Physiol. (London)*, **115**, 101.

Scalzi, H. A. and Price, H. M. (1971). 'The arrangement and sensory innervation of the intrafusal fibers in the feline muscle spindle.' *J. Ultrastruct. Res.*, **36**, 375.

Smorto, M. P. and Basmajian, J. V. (1972). In *Clinical Electroneurography*. Baltimore; Williams and Wilkins.

Spencer, P. S. and Schaumburg, A. H. (1973). 'An ultrastructural study of the inner core of the Pacinian corpuscle.' *J. Neurocytol.*, **2**, 217.

Swash, M. and Fox, K. P. (1972). 'Muscle spindle innervation in man.' *J. Anat.*, **112**, 61.

Thoenen, H. (1972). 'Neuronally mediated enzyme induction in adrenergic neurons and adrenal chromaffin cells.' *Biochem. Soc. Symp.*, **36**, 3.

Thomas, P. K. (1963). 'The connective tissue of peripheral nerve: an electron microscope study.' *J. Anat.*, **97**, 35.

Tomonaga, M. and Sluga, E. (1970). 'Zur Ultrastruktur der π-Granula.' *Acta Neuropath. (Berlin)*, **15**, 56.

Vandenheuvel, F. A. (1968). 'Structural studies of biological membranes: the structure of myelin.' *Ann. N.Y. Acad. Sci.*, **122**, 57.

Vizoso, A. D. and Young, J. Z. (1948). 'The internode length and fibre diameter in developing and regenerating nerves.' *J. Anat.*, **82**, 110.

Waller, A. (1850). 'Experiments on the section of the glossopharyngeal and hypoglossal nerves of the frog and observations of the alterations produced thereby in the structure of their primitive fibres.' *Phil. Trans. Roy. Soc.*, **140**, 423.

Warwick, R. and Williams, P. L. (1973). In *Gray's Anatomy*, 35th edn. Edinburgh; Longman.

Webster, H. de F. and Spiro, D. (1960). 'Phase and electron microscopic studies of experimental demyelination. I. Variations in myelin sheath contour in normal guinea pig sciatic nerve.' *J. Neuropath. Exp. Neurol.*, **19**, 42.

Weiss, P. and Hiscoe, H. B. (1948). 'Experiments on the mechanism of nerve growth.' *J. Exp. Zool.*, **107**, 315.

Weller, R. O. (1967). 'An electron microscopic study of hypertrophic neuropathy of Dejerine and Sottas.' *J. Neurol. Neurosurg. Psychiat.*, **30**, 111.

Weller, R. O. and Das Gupta, T. K. (1968). 'Experimental hypertrophic neuropathy: an electron microscope study.' *J. Neurol. Neurosurg. Psychiat.*, **31**, 34.

Weller, R. O. and Herzog, I. (1970). 'Schwann cell lysosomes in hypertrophic neuropathy and in normal human nerves.' *Brain*, **93**, 347.

REFERENCES

Williams, P. L. and Landon, D. N. (1963). 'Paranodal apparatus of peripheral myelinated nerve fibres of mammals.' *Nature (London)*, **198,** 670.

Williams, P. L. and Wendell-Smith, C. P. (1971). 'Some additional parametric variations between peripheral nerve fibre populations.' *J. Anat.*, **109,** 505.

Wisniewski, H., Terry, R. D. and Hirano, A. (1970). 'Neurofibrillary pathology.' *J. Neuropath. Exp. Neurol.*, **29,** 163.

Zaimis, E. and Maclagan, J. (1974). 'General physiology and pharmacology of neuromuscular transmission.' In *Disorders of Voluntary Muscle,* 3rd edn. Ed. by J. N. Walton. Edinburgh; Churchill Livingstone.

4

General Pathology of Peripheral Nerves

INTRODUCTION

Normal function of the peripheral nervous system depends upon an intact brain and spinal cord in addition to the functional and structural integrity of the peripheral nerve components. The nervous system as a whole is so integrated that defects in one portion may have widespread effects throughout the whole system. It is advisable, therefore, when discussing the general pathology of the peripheral nervous system, to look also at disease processes in the central nervous system that affect peripheral nerve function.

The peripheral nervous system and its central connections can be viewed from several aspects.

Input. Motor neurones in the anterior horns of the spinal cord and in cranial nerve nuclei are influenced by other neurones in the central nervous system. Terminal boutons from these neurones form synapses on dendrites and the cell body of the motor neurones (*Figure 26*). Some boutons are excitatory, while others are inhibitory. The input into motor neurones may be disordered when upper motor neurones and the corticospinal tracts degenerate as in many cases of motor neurone disease (Liversedge and Campbell, 1974). Disturbances of input occur if demyelinating plaques of multiple sclerosis involve the corticospinal or extrapyramidal tracts, and many of the effects of Parkinson's disease can be attributed to disordered input into lower motor neurones.

Most of the input into dorsal root ganglion sensory neurones is mediated through the axons connecting the neurones with the periphery. Disorders of sensory input are seen, therefore, when the end-organs or the peripheral nerve axons are diseased.

Neurones. The cell soma of motor and sensory neurones contains the nucleus and the perinuclear cytoplasm in which most of the cell organelles are produced and where protein synthesis for the cell and its processes occurs. If the neuronal cell body is destroyed, its dendrites and axon do not survive. There are a number of different disease processes which result in the loss of

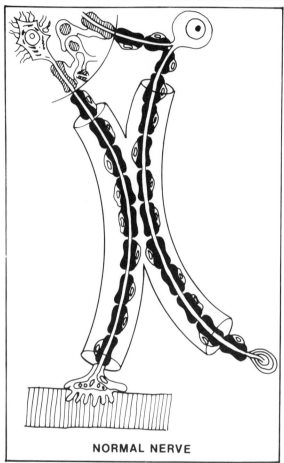

NORMAL NERVE

Fig. 26. Diagram to show the relationship of motor and sensory neurones with their myelinated fibres and end-organs. Oligodendroglia myelinate the axons in the spinal cord and Schwann cells myelinate the peripheral nerve fibres

motor neurones of the spinal cord and the brain stem. Some have a genetic basis or an unknown aetiology and fall into the category of motor neurone disease (Liversedge and Campbell, 1974). In these diseases there is loss of motor neurones with consequent muscle atrophy (amyotrophy). There is selective loss of motor neurones in certain virus diseases, particularly poliomyelitis. Less selective damage to the spinal cord from trauma, ischaemia, etc., may result in loss of motor neurones (Hughes, 1966). A number of sensory neuropathies are marked by a reduction in posterior root ganglion cells (Brain and Walton, 1969), and virus infections, such as herpes zoster, damage the dorsal root ganglion (Dayan, Ogul and Graveson, 1972). Degeneration of posterior roots or ganglia is accompanied by degeneration of fibres in the posterior columns of the spinal cord.

Functional integrity of the neurone is as important as structural integrity,

INTRODUCTION

and in some neuropathies the cell bodies are preserved but the distal ends of
the nerves degenerate. The term 'dying back' neuropathy is used for this
condition and it is seen in certain toxic neuropathies, e.g. acrylamide (Fullerton
and Barnes, 1966; Prineas, 1969b) and organophosphorus poisoning
(Cavanagh, 1964, 1973; Prineas, 1969a). The distal ends of large-diameter
nerve fibres innervating the foot muscles are most severely affected in 'dying
back' neuropathies. At present it is not clear whether the degenerative process
is induced by direct action of the toxin upon the axon terminals or whether it is
the result of toxic damage to the whole neurone (Prineas, 1969a). Cavanagh
and Chen (1971) demonstrated inhibition of protein synthesis in neurone cell
bodies before the onset of distal degeneration in a 'dying back' neuropathy.
This may be sufficient to cause the distal degeneration of long, large-diameter
axons. Bradley and Williams (1973), on the other hand, found no significant
decrease in axoplasmic flow in triorthocresyl phosphate, acrylamide or
vincristine neuropathies.

Axons. The dependence of the axon upon the cell body for supply of
nutrients, cell organelles and proteins is emphasized by the degeneration of the
axon that occurs if it is severed from the cell body. The nerve terminals also
degenerate following nerve section and denervated muscle fibres atrophy.

Axonal degeneration occurs in many peripheral neuropathies, including
ischaemic neuropathies (Dyck, Conn and Okazaki, 1972) and nerves locally
infiltrated by tumour. Severe segmental demyelinating neuropathies may be
accompanied by axonal degeneration (Bradley and Jennekens, 1971).

Although regeneration occurs, it is slow and in many cases it is only partly
effective, as the end-organs have degenerated and the regenerating neurites do
not always re-establish the correct connections.

Myelin sheath. Normal conduction of the impulse along myelinated nerve
fibres depends upon an intact myelin sheath. If the myelin is deficient, the
conduction velocity of the impulse is reduced and it may fail altogether
(Thomas, 1971). Demyelination of the axons may occur in the central nervous
system in multiple sclerosis, with little subsequent remyelination (Adams and
Leibowitz, 1972). In peripheral nerves demyelination occurs in a segmental
distribution (segmental demyelination) and the axon remains intact; each
segment is the distance between consecutive nodes of Ranvier and represents
the length of nerve fibre myelinated by a single Schwann cell.

Unless the demyelination is severe, the axons remain intact, the end-organs
do not degenerate and there is little muscle atrophy. Remyelination often
occurs very promptly and recovery of neurological function may be complete.

In chronic, recurrent demyelinating neuropathies there is progressive proliferation of Schwann cells and the formation of imbricated 'onion-bulb'
cellular whorls producing the classical appearance of hypertrophic
neuropathy.

Integrity of the nerve endings. The release of acetyl choline or
catecholamines from nerve endings is the basis of neural transmission to other
neurones or effector organs such as muscle. When the nerve endings
degenerate following axonal section, neuronal death or 'dying back'
neuropathy, neural transmission ceases. Functional disorders of neuromuscular transmission can be induced by tetanus or botulinum toxin,
with subsequent sprouting of nerve terminals (Duchen, 1971). Similar
pathological changes have been described in myasthenia gravis in man

63

(Brownell, Oppenheimer and Spalding, 1972), where there is a disorder of neuromuscular transmission.

The main pathological features of axonal degeneration and segmental demyelination that are seen in peripheral nerves will be described in further detail.

Chronic peripheral neuropathies may show hypertrophic changes with onion-bulb formation and this phenomenon will also be described in this chapter. Many of the structures involved in diseases of the peripheral nervous system are only available for histological study at post-mortem; this applies particularly to spinal cord, dorsal root ganglia and nerve roots. However, some indication of pathological mechanism involving these structures may be obtained from the histological study of biopsies or autopsy specimens of more peripheral parts of the nerve.

PATHOLOGICAL REACTIONS IN PERIPHERAL NERVES

AXONAL DEGENERATION AND REGENERATION

Axonal degeneration

There is an element of axonal degeneration in almost all peripheral neuropathies, even those that are predominantly segmental demyelinating lesions. The course of axonal degeneration and regeneration has been extensively studied by light microscopy (Cajal, 1928), by histochemical techniques (Adams, 1965; Hallpike, 1972) and by electron microscopy (Nathaniel and Pease, 1963 a,b; Morris, Hudson and Weddell, 1972a–d).

Most experimenters have used the technique of nerve crush to study axonal degeneration and regeneration, for if the nerve trunk is completely severed, continuity of connective tissue elements is lost and regeneration is inhibited and less effective. Some retrograde axonal degeneration occurs in the very terminal portion of the proximal nerve stump following a crush (Morris *et al.*, 1972a), but the major degenerative changes are seen in the axon and myelin sheaths of the distal stump. Changes are observed initially in the proximal part of the distal stump of the nerve near the site of injury and gradually progress towards the distal end of the severed portion of nerve. By 24 h after injury most myelinated and non-myelinated fibres show extensive degeneration (Thomas, King and Phelps, 1972).

Within the first two hours after axon crush or section the distal and proximal stumps retract (Morgan-Hughes and Engel, 1968). The Schwann cell also reacts during this early period, with widening of the Schmidt–Lantermann incisures in the myelin sheath near the focus of damage and retraction of myelin from nodes of Ranvier (Williams and Hall, 1971). These changes gradually spread along the distal stump of the nerve. Acid phosphatase activity is detected in the distal stump near the site of injury within 2–3 h; it is localized ultrastructurally to dilated smooth membrane vesicles (Holtzman and Novikoff, 1965) and gradually over the next 12 h the enzyme activity spreads distally. Other ultrastructural changes that are seen in the axons of the distal stump at this time probably reflect the cessation of normal axonal flow and the disintegration of cell organelles. Within the first 24 h there is focal

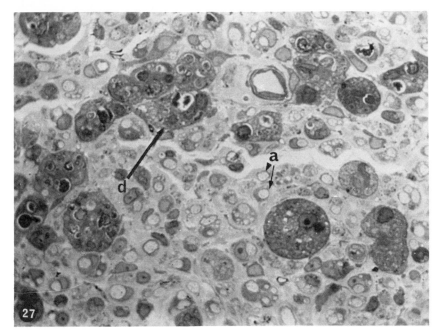

Fig. 27. T.S. peripheral nerve at the site of nerve injury 21 days after damage. Macrophages and Schwann cells contain myelin debris (d). Regenerating axon sprouts, as yet unmyelinated, are also seen (a). 1 μm Araldite section stained with toluidine blue. × 744

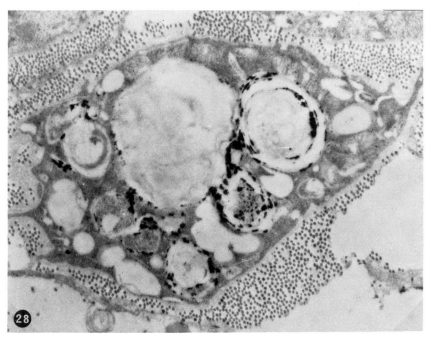

Fig. 28. Ten days axonal degeneration. Acid phosphatase activity (black deposit) is associated with the breakdown of myelin debris within Schwann cell vacuoles. Electron micrograph: Gomori technique × 9800 (Courtesy of Br. J. Exp. Pathol.)

accumulation of mitochondria, microtubules, dilated vesicles and degenerate organelles within swollen portions of axons and at nodes of Ranvier (Ballin and Thomas, 1969c). Subsequently the axon fragments (Cajal, 1928), and becomes shrunken and densely staining in electron micrographs. As the axon breaks up, the myelin sheath becomes disrupted and forms globules within the Schwann cytoplasm (*Figure 27*). Ultrastructural studies have shown that myelin end-loops peel off the axon at the nodes of Ranvier and the sheath lamellae split along the interperiod line (Ballin and Thomas, 1969c).

The fragmented axon and myelin debris are broken down within lysosomal vacuoles in Schwann cells (*Figure 28*) and to some extent within macrophages which migrate into the nerve during early stages of degeneration (Weller and Mellick, 1966). Loss of basic protein from the myelin 24 h after nerve crush is one of the earliest chemical changes in the degenerating myelin (Hallpike, 1972). Significant increases in lysosomal enzymes related to myelin debris do not occur until 6–7 days after crush (Weller and Mellick, 1966; Hallpike, 1972). It is at this time that the major chemical changes occur in the myelin lipids, with the formation of sudanophilic cholesterol esters (Adams, 1965).

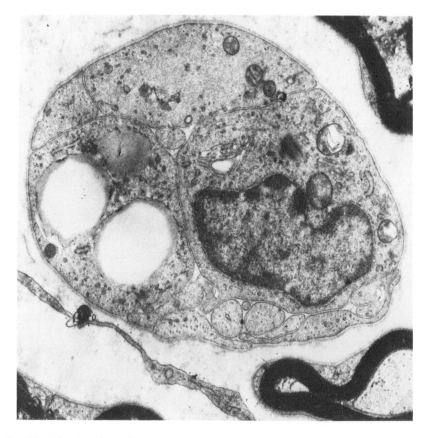

Fig. 29. T.S. of a band of Büngner. The axon has degenerated; the Schwann cell and its processes containing lipid droplets remain surrounded by a basement membrane. Electron micrograph × 10 000

Initially the globules of myelin debris are birefringent and retain their lamellated ultrastructure, but as the cholesterol becomes esterified to cholesterol esters, the lipid debris loses its birefringent properties and is seen as amorphous osmiophilic lipid in electron micrographs (*Figure 29*). At this stage the lipid droplets stain strongly with Sudan dyes and Oil red O and are Marchi-positive. During the second week after nerve crush much of the myelin debris is removed from the nerve and regenerative features become more prominent.

Degeneration of the distal part of the axons in 'dying back' neuropathies bears many similarities to axon degeneration following crush, except that the early ultrastructural changes are spread over a much longer period. In the 'dying back' neuropathy induced by triorthocresyl phosphates there is accumulation of smooth membrane-bound vesicles (Prineas, 1969a), whereas neurofilaments tend to be more prominent in the axons in acrylamide neuropathy (Prineas, 1969b).

Nerve regeneration

Fine axon sprouts (*Figure 27*) grow from the proximal stumps of the severed axons into the distal stump of the nerve where the Schwann cells have multiplied and formed longitudinal bands (bands of Büngner) (Bradley and Asbury, 1970). As the regenerating axons grow distally, many become myelinated and some may eventually re-establish peripheral connections (*Figure 30*).

Within 48 h of injury the terminal end of the proximal axon stump swells to form a regeneraing end-bulb full of cytoplasm and organelles (Morris *et al.*, 1972c). Some bulbs are very large, e.g. 800 μm long and 9 μm in diameter for an axon 4 μm in diameter (Kreutzberg and Schubert, 1971). After 6 days several axon sprouts, 1–1·5 μm in diameter, grow from each end-bulb towards the distal stump of the nerve, where the Schwann cells have started to divide and proliferate despite the myelin debris in their cytoplasm (Bradley and Asbury, 1970). The Schwann cells of the distal stump form long bands of Büngner which act as guidelines for the growth of axon sprouts. At first the regenerating axons are clustered together in a similar way to the non-myelinated fibres (Morris *et al.*, 1972b), but by 7–10 days the clusters become looser as individual axons are separated and invaginated into the surface of Schwann cells. Several axons may be invaginated into one Schwann cell but gradually the supernumerary axons are suppressed and a 1:1 axon–Schwann cell relationship is re-established (Nathaniel and Pease, 1963b).

Axon sprouts from myelinated fibres acquire myelin sheaths formed from Schwann cell membrane in a similar way to primary myelination in developing nerves. The small axons have thin myelin sheaths which increase in thickness as the axon diameter increases. Regenerating axon sprouts from a single nerve fibre appear to remain closely associated with each other in a cluster of small myelinated fibres surrounded by the same basement membrane. Small clusters are often seen in peripheral neuropathies, especially when there is repeated axon degeneration and regeneration (Schröder, 1968). Thomas (1970) found that normally after one nerve crush only one axon sprout from each myelinated axon became myelinated but after multiple periodic nerve crushes

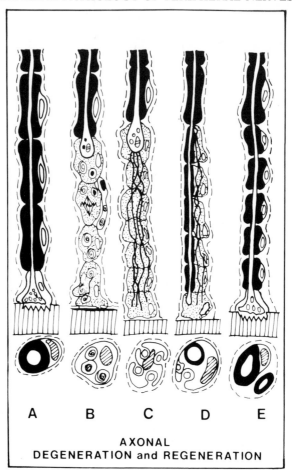

Fig. 30. Diagram summarizing the events occurring during axonal degeneration and regeneration. A. Normal nerve. B. Seven days after axonal damage; Schwann cells containing axon and myelin debris have divided to form bands of Büngner. C. Axon sprouts grow from the swollen end bulb of the proximal axon. D. An axon becomes myelinated. E. Connection with the end-organ is re-established; regenerated internodes are short.

many more axon sprouts became myelinated, producing a myriad of clusters of small myelinated fibres.

Regenerating axons grow distally at between 2—5 mm day^{-1}, depending upon the species, but in many instances the axons may not achieve their former peripheral connections, in which case the myelinated fibres remain small. Even the fibres that do re-establish connections do not usually attain full maturity of axon diameter and myelin sheath thickness (Cragg and Thomas, 1964).

Axon regeneration may occur in 'dying back' neuropathies induced by toxic chemicals such as acrylamide, especially if the toxin is no longer administered (Fullerton and Barnes, 1966).

Degeneration and regeneration in non-myelinated axons has received less attention than the more easily detected events involving myelinated fibres. Dyck and Hopkins (1972) studied the effects of crushing the cervical sympathetic trunk in the rat, where 99 per cent of the axons are non-myelinated and are less than 1 μm in diameter (mode, 0·4 μm). Degeneration was well advanced at 69 h and followed a very similar pattern of axonal fragmentation to that seen in myelinated axons. Regeneration was detectable by 5 days, although at 15 weeks most of the axons were still small (mode, 0·25 μm). Nerve conduction in the sympathetic trunk returned by 10 days and had reached normal values by 30–40 days (Hopkins and Lambert, 1972). Degeneration of non-myelinated fibres in human peripheral neuropathies is seen especially in diabetes (Thomas, 1973), amyloid (Dyck and Lambert, 1969), Fabry's disease (Bischoff *et al.*, 1968), familial dysautonomia or Riley–Day syndrome (Aguayo, Nair and Bray, 1971). Non-myelinated fibres and ganglion cells in the autonomic nervous system fail to develop or are destroyed in animals treated with nerve growth factor antiserum (Aguayo, Martin and Bray, 1972).

Remote effects of axonal degeneration and regeneration

There are two main effects to be considered under this heading: chromatolysis of the neurone and neurogenic atrophy of muscle.

Chromatolysis

Chromatolysis occurs if an axon is severed near the neurone and especially if the axon is repeatedly injured. Most sequential studies have been done on the facial or hypoglossal nerve (Kreutzberg, 1972) where the nerves have been damaged close to the neurone cell body.

The earliest changes involving the neurones are seen at 2–4 days after severing the facial nerve. Microglia proliferate around the motor neurones, and by 4 days microglial processes have displaced about 60 per cent of the synapses from the neuronal cell surface (Blinzinger and Kreutzberg, 1968). At about the same time as the loss of most of its afferent connections the neurone starts to swell. This is the onset of chromatolysis, and at 2 days the neurone may be twice its original volume. The Nissl substance, consisting of granular endoplasmic reticulum and polyribosomes, is dispersed to the edge of the cell (Cervós-Navarro, 1962) and the centre of the cell loses much of its staining. As the cell swells, the nucleus and nucleolus become eccentrically placed in the neurone (*Figure 31*).

For many years chromatolysis was thought to be a degenerative process, but as there is a very marked increase in RNA and protein synthesis during this period, it is now considered to be a regenerative process (Kreutzberg, 1972). The neurone remains in a highly active metabolic state during the phase of axon regeneration, which may last for several months.

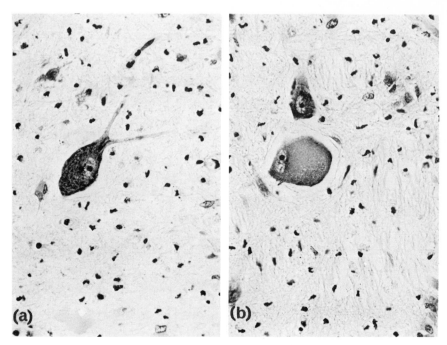

Fig. 31. Chromatolysis. (a) Normal anterior horn cell with abundant Nissl substance. (b) Chromatolytic anterior horn cell with an eccentric nucleus, and swollen pale cytoplasm. Nissl stain; × 294

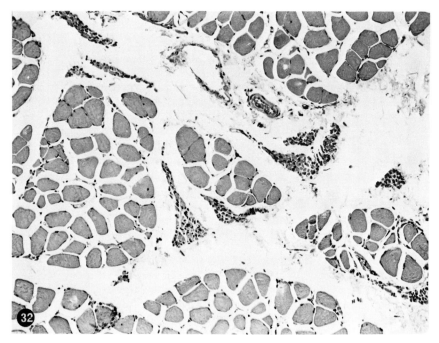

Fig. 32. T.S. muscle: denervation atrophy. Groups of small atrophic fibres are mixed with normal muscle fibres. H. and E. stain; × 120

Neurogenic atrophy of muscle

Soon after the axon degenerates, the muscle end-plate that it supplies also degenerates and the muscle fibre atrophies. If denervation of the muscle is extensive, there is group atrophy of muscle fibres (*Figure 32*). In many chronic neuropathies, where axons degenerate a few at a time, there may be collateral sprouting of remaining axons and the effect upon the muscle is less dramatic. These cases often show scattered small angulated Type 1 and Type 2 muscle fibres in muscle biopsies.

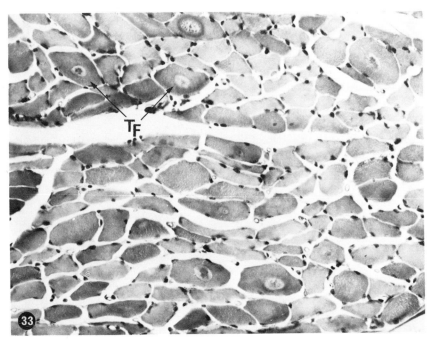

Fig. 33. T.S. muscle. Target fibres (TF) in motor neurone disease. *Gomori trichrome stain;* × 240

Another histological change in muscle that is associated with long-standing denervation and perhaps reinnervation is the presence of target fibres (*Figure 33*) (Dubowitz and Brooke, 1973). They resemble central core disease in oxidative enzyme histochemical preparations with a central zone devoid of enzyme activity and mitochondria; disorganization of the myofibrils is seen electron microscopically. An intermediate zone of myofibrillar disarray separates the central zone of the target fibres from the more normal peripheral parts of the fibre.

Detection of axonal degeneration and regeneration in peripheral nerve biopsies

Following traumatic section or acute infarction of the nerve, many of the nerve fibres are at the same stage of degeneration or regeneration at the same time (*Figure 27*). In many neuropathies, however, individual fibres are damaged at different times, so it is important to be able to recognize different stages of degeneration and regeneration in the same section of nerve. Extensive nerve fibre loss may be observed in severe long-standing peripheral neuropathies; these changes may be obvious, but detection of less extensive changes may require careful quantitation (Dyck *et al.,* 1968).

The early stages of axonal degeneration are detected most frequently in the acute stages of neuropathies, e.g. Guillain–Barré polyneuropathy, or following trauma or infarction. In frozen sections sudanophilic globular lipid droplets of myelin breakdown products are seen in Schwann cells and macrophages; acid phosphatase is also associated with these cells. Axon stains in paraffin sections reveal fragmentation of axons. Individual fibres in teased preparations show myelin breakdown throughout the fibre distal to the site of damage (cf. segmental demyelination). One-μm epoxy resin sections and electron microscopy reveal the degenerative process in more detail, and if only occasional fibres are degenerating, they are usually more easily detected in these preparations than in paraffin sections.

Regeneration in peripheral nerves can be detected both in the very early stages and in nerves where regeneration has taken place in the past. Silver-stained longitudinal paraffin sections may reveal fine axon sprouts distal to the point of injury and swollen axon balloons (regeneration growth cones) just proximal to the injury.

In teased preparations fibres in the early stages of regeneration have thin axons and thin myelin sheaths. At a later stage, when axons and myelin have almost regained their original dimensions, the regenerated fibres in an adult can be detected because the internodes are much shorter in length than normal nerves. When the Schwann cells divide following degeneration of the axons, they re-establish their embryonic length of about 300 μm. Thus, even the large 10 μm diameter regenerated myelinated fibres may have an internodal length of 400 μm instead of 1000 μm or more (Fullerton *et al.,* 1965).

In 1 μm epoxy resin sections and electron microscopy the cellular detail is usually much better preserved. Axon balloons (regeneration cones) may be prominent; they are seen in transverse sections as swollen axons stuffed with organelles and with a rather thin myelin sheath stretched around the outside. In longitudinal sections the balloons are seen to be bulbous swellings at the end of the proximal stump of the axon. Axons in the early stages of regeneration will be small and the axon diameter:myelin sheath thickness ratio will be approximately normal (cf. myelination following segmental demyelination where there is axon:myelin disproportion).

Chronic peripheral neuropathies, particularly those with recurrent episodes of axonal degeneration, often show a reduction in the large-diameter fibres and a relative increase in small fibres (Weller, Bruckner and Chamberlain, 1970). Many of the small myelinated fibres may be in clusters (*Figure 34*) surrounded by a common basement membrane and represent a group of regeneration sprouts from a single larger axon (Ochoa and Mair, 1969b; Morris *et al.,* 1972b). When the nerve is severely affected, most of the myelinated fibres are lost (*Figure 35*). The large-diameter myelinated fibres usually disappear from the nerve before the small-diameter fibres and finally the non-myelinated fibres are lost. The latter are really only well studied and quantified by electron microscopy. In a very severely affected nerve only the Schwann cells may

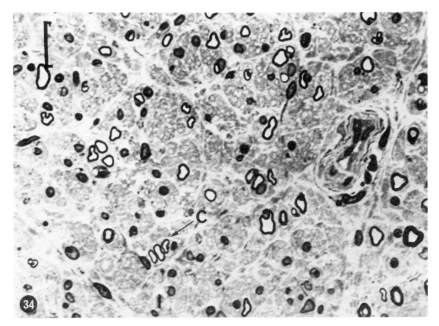

Fig. 34. Chronic peripheral neuropathy with axonal degeneration. There is loss of large myelinated fibres. Clusters of myelinated regenerating axon sprouts (C) are seen. Numerous non-myelinated fibres are preserved. 1 μm Araldite section stained with toluidine blue. × 700 (Courtesy of J. Neurol. Neurosurg. Psychiat.)

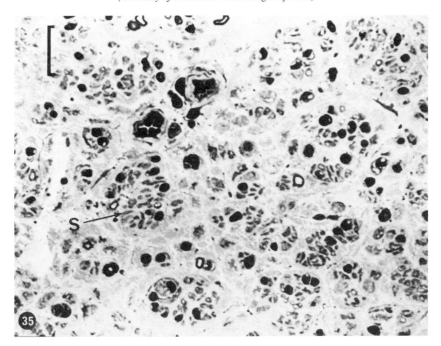

Fig. 35. Chronic peripheral neuropathy. There is an almost total loss of myelinated and non-myelinated fibres. Cords of Schwann cells (S) remain devoid of axons. 1 μm Araldite section toluidine blue stained. × 700 (Courtesy of J. Neurol. Neurosurg. Psychiat.)

73

remain as rather atrophic bands. The detection of axonal degeneration and regeneration in the 'dying-back' neuropathies is best seen in thick sections of muscle stained for axons or myelin (Cavanagh, Passingham and Vogt, 1964).

SEGMENTAL DEMYELINATION

About 30 years after Waller's (1850) classical description of axonal degeneration, Gombault (1880) described segmental demyelination in the nerves of guinea-pigs suffering from chronic lead intoxication. The axons remain intact in segmental demyelination but short segments of myelin break down along the length of individual nerve fibres. Each segment represents the length of one Schwann cell and its myelin sheath. Several consecutive segments along the same nerve may be affected, producing much longer lengths of demyelination. In many cases remyelination begins soon after demyelination has occurred. As the axons remain intact, there is little wasting of muscles and, with the completion of remyelination, recovery from a purely segmental demyelinating neuropathy is virtually complete. Some axonal degeneration is usually seen, however, especially in severe segmental demyelinating neuropathies.

There are two basic types of segmental demyelination. (1) *Primary segmental demyelination*, where a metabolic disturbance in the Schwann cell results in breakdown of the myelin sheath by the Schwann cell itself. (2) *Allergic segmental demyelination* due to delayed hypersensitivity reaction (cell-mediated immune reaction), where the myelin sheath is broken down by macrophages with lymphocytes in close attendance. Schwann cells may also play a role in the breakdown of the sheath, but this is variable.

Primary segmental demyelination (*Figure 36*)

This type of segmental demyelination occurs particularly in diphtheritic neuropathy (Fisher and Adams, 1956; Cavanagh and Jacobs, 1964), lead neuropathy (Fullerton, 1966; Lampert and Schochet, 1968) and diabetic neuropathy (Ballin and Thomas, 1968). It appears to be due to interference with Schwann cell metabolism, especially protein synthesis (Pleasure, Feldman and Prockop, 1973). Schwann cells seem to be more vulnerable to ischaemia than axons, so segmental demyelination is seen in the more mild forms of ischaemic neuropathy (Eames and Lange, 1967) and rheumatoid neuropathy (Weller *et al.*, 1970). More severe damage to the nerves in these neuropathies results in axonal degeneration.

Diphtheritic neuropathy is the most commonly used experimental model for primary segmental demyelination. Experimental animals injected with appropriate amounts of toxin either systemically (Cavanagh and Jacobs, 1964) or intraneurally (Jacobs, Cavanagh and Mellick, 1966), show clinical signs of a peripheral neuropathy after 5–21 days, depending upon the experimental animal. Although segmental demyelination occurs at the same time as the onset of neurological signs, the effect of the toxin on the Schwann cells takes place within the first hour after injection and after that time cannot be modified by antitoxin (Cavanagh and Jacobs, 1964).

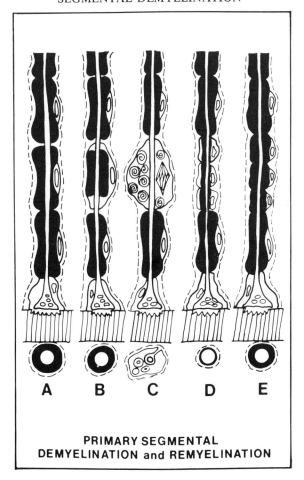

PRIMARY SEGMENTAL
DEMYELINATION and REMYELINATION

Fig. 36. Diagram to summarize the events occurring in primary segmental demyelination and remyelination. A. Normal nerve. B. Early segmental demyelination: retraction of paranodal myelin with widening of the nodal gap. C. Destruction of myelin sheath and Schwann cell mitosis. D, E. Remyelination: intercalated short segments

The earliest signs of segmental demyelination are usually seen at the node of Ranvier (*Figure 37*). There is retraction of myelin from the node with detachment of myelin end-loops and widening of the nodal gap (Allt and Cavanagh, 1969). In the smaller-diameter myelinated fibres the myelin may break down throughout the whole internode, whereas there may only be paranodal demyelination in the larger fibres. Once the nodal gap reaches some 100 μm, however, the whole length of the internodal myelin usually breaks down (Cavanagh and Jacobs, 1964).

Disruption of the myelin sheath is primarily by the Schwann cell which originally produced it. At the node the myelin end-bulbs are retracted and the myelin fragments are degraded within lysosomal vacuoles. No direct involvement of lysosomal enzymes has been observed in the early disruption of

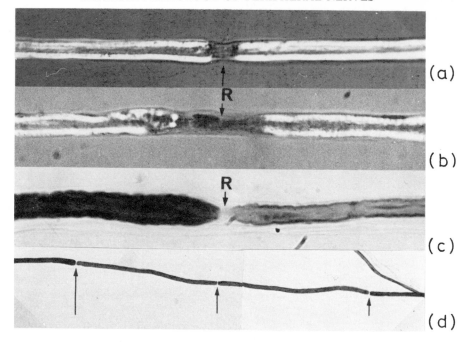

Fig. 37. Teased fibres in primary segmental demyelination and remyelination. (a) Early segmental demyelination: widening of the nodal gap (R). NADH-TR stain and polarized light. ×640. (Courtesy of Brain.) (b) Further widening of the nodal gap (R). Schwann cytoplasm and axon stained by NADH-TR technique occupy the gap between the myelin segments. Polarized light. ×640. (Courtesy of Brain.) (c) Remyelination: a thinly myelinated, remyelinating segment is seen to the right of the node of Ranvier (R). Osmium-fixed nerve. ×790. (d) Remyelination: short remyelinated segments 400 μm in length (normal~1200 μm). Osmium-fixed. (Nodes of Ranvier marked by arrows.) ×100

myelin at the node (Weller and Nester, 1972). But disruption of the internodal myelin sheath in smaller fibres may be initiated by lysosomal enzymes (Weller, 1965); so that the myelin sheath is split longitudinally and retracted from around the axon, leaving the latter undamaged. Chemical changes in the disrupted myelin follow a similar sequence to that seen after axonal degeneration, with the formation of sudanophilic cholesterol ester droplets and subsequent removal of the lipid from the nerve. One major difference in the histological picture is that an intact axon remains associated with the Schwann cell throughout.

Allergic segmental demyelination *(Figure 38)*

There are certain peripheral neuropathies, most notably the Landry–Guillain–Barré syndrome (Prineas, 1972) and experimental allergic neuritis (Waksman and Adams, 1955; Ballin and Thomas, 1969a), where there is lymphocyte and macrophage infiltration of the nerve fascicles and segmental demyelination. If the neuropathy is severe, axonal degeneration may be extensive. Clinically, the Guillain–Barré syndrome (Prineas, 1972) presents as a

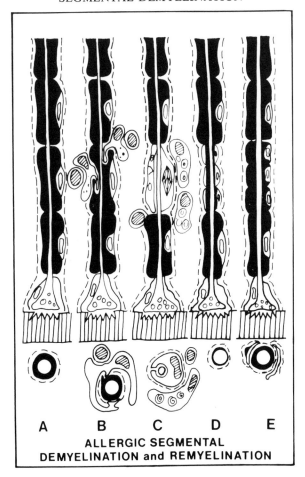

Fig. 38. Diagram to summarize allergic segmental demyelination and remyelination. A. Normal fibre. B. Demyelination; macrophages are stripping the myelin sheath. Associated lymphocytes are also shown. C. Schwann cell mitosis. D, E. Remyelination

motor neuropathy often 2–4 weeks after a viral infection. It may progress for 2–4 weeks and then the patient usually recovers virtually completely over the next 3–6 months. The anterior spinal roots are often most severely affected.

Experimental allergic neuritis (EAN) has many similar pathological features to the Guillain–Barré syndrome (Prineas, 1972). It is produced by the intra-cutaneous injection of emulsified peripheral nerve myelin together with Freund's adjuvant (Waksman and Adams, 1955; Astrom, Webster and Arnason, 1968; Ballin and Thomas, 1969a). Allergic demyelination in the CNS (experimental allergic encephalomyelitis) can be induced by an injection of emulsified CNS myelin with Freund's adjuvant, or just with the basic protein component of myelin mixed with Freund's adjuvant (Leibowitz, 1972).

The onset of signs of peripheral neuropathy in EAN occurs 2–3 weeks after the injection and is accompanied by segmental demyelination. Ultrastructural studies have shown that macrophages, in the presence of lymphocytes,

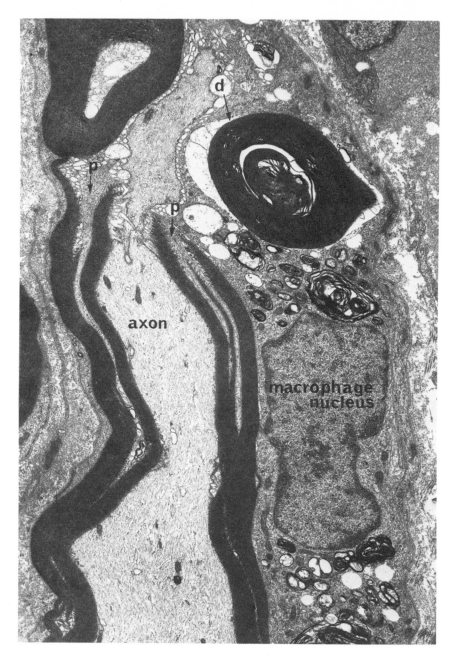

Fig. 39. Allergic segmental demyelination in a rabbit posterior root with experimental allergic neuritis. Macrophage processes (p) are stripping the myelin from the axon at a node of Ranvier. Myelin debris (d) is seen in the macrophage cytoplasm. × 8700 (Courtesy of Dr G. Allt and J. Neurocytol.)

penetrate the basement membrane around intact nerve fibres and displace the Schwann cytoplasm from the myelin sheath (*Figure 39*). Subsequent stripping of the myelin sheath and dissolution of the myelin is performed chiefly by the macrophages in the presence of lymphocytes (Wisniewski, Prineas and Raine, 1969). Macrophages may attack the myelin at the node of Ranvier or in its internodal portion. The role of Schwann cells in the demyelinating process is variable (Ballin and Thomas, 1969a): in some cases the Schwann cell appears to play no part in the breakdown of the myelin sheath, whereas in others it plays a major role. The association of lymphocytes with the macrophages that are destroying the myelin sheath, and the finding that EAN can be transferred to other animals by sensitized lymphocytes (Astrom and Waksman, 1962), strongly suggests that EAN is a cell-mediated immune response.

There are two features of the Guillain–Barré syndrome that suggest its immunological nature and its close relationship with EAN. First, the histological and ultrastructural features of demyelination are very similar (Prineas, 1972). Second, there is specific lymphocyte stimulation by peripheral nerve basic protein in patients with Guillain–Barré syndrome (Knowles *et al.*, 1968), which emphasizes the cellular hypersensitivity to myelin in this disease. So far, however, the exact aetiology of the hypersensitivity is uncertain (Bradley, 1974), but it may be a virus-induced auto-immune reaction. This suggestion is supported by the close similarity of the pathological reactions in the peripheral nerves of Guillain–Barré syndrome (Prineas, 1972) and Marek's disease, a proven virus disease of chickens (Prineas and Wright, 1972).

Remyelination

A similar pattern of remyelination occurs following primary and allergic segmental demyelination (*Figures 36* and *38*). Furthermore, the mode of myelin sheath formation resembles in many respects the process of myelination in developing nerves (Allt, 1969; Ballin and Thomas, 1969b). Following demyelination the involved Schwann cells divide. Many mitoses are seen 1–2 days after demyelination has commenced in diphtheritic neuropathy (Jacobs *et al.*, 1966) at a time when myelin breakdown is actively proceeding. There is a striking increase in nuclear population within the nerve during the subsequent 10 days. Some of these cells are macrophages but many are Schwann cells which migrate to remyelinate the demyelinated segments. Patterns of remyelination depend upon the extent to which the particular internode is demyelinated. If there is very little nodal gap widening, less than 15 μm, then the gap may be remyelinated by extension of the internodal myelin back to the mode of Ranvier (Allt, 1969). When the nodal gap is wider, up to 40 μm, a single Schwann cell migrates into the gap to remyelinate the axon and form a short intercalated segment (Ballin and Thomas, 1969b). Breakdown of myelin throughout the whole internode occurs if paranodal demyelination spreads to involve more than half the internode. In this case remyelination of the whole segment is effected by two or three Schwann cells each reverting to the original embryonic length of 300–400 μm (*Figure 37*).

Electron microscope studies have shown how the large-diameter demyelinated axons become invaginated into Schwann cells, the mesaxon elongates in a spiral around the axon and then becomes compacted to form myelin. Gradually the myelin sheath increases in thickness until the myelin:axon ratio reaches a more or less normal value. Many structural irregularities and bizarre configurations have been observed during remyelination (Ballin and Thomas, 1969b).

Remyelination seems to follow the same basic pattern in many neuropathies where segmental demyelination is a prominent feature, but the speed of remyelination and the effectiveness of the remyelination differ. For example, remyelination in experimental allergic neuritis and diphtheritic neuropathy usually begin within about 2 weeks of demyelination (Ballin and Thomas, 1969b; Weller and Nester, 1972), whereas in some chronic demyelinating neuropathies (cf. hypertrophic neuropathy) and in certain metabolic diseases of Schwann cells, e.g. sulphatide lipidosis (metachromatic leukodystrophy), the myelin sheaths remain very thin and may never regain their normal thickness.

Detection of segmental demyelination and remyelination in peripheral nerves

The best way to detect segmental demyelination and remyelination in the individual nerve fibres is to examine teased preparations (*Figure 37*). Osmium tetroxide can be used to stain the myelin, or, if enzyme and lipid histochemistry is required, the teased preparations can be examined by polarized light (Weller and Nester, 1972; see Chapter 2). Retraction of the myelin from the node of Ranvier with widening of the nodal gap is usually the earliest change seen in segmental demyelination. The axon retains its continuity across the gap in the myelin sheath, which is also filled with Schwann cytoplasm. At a later stage the myelin may break down throughout the whole internode and the demyelinated axon traverses the whole segment surrounded by Schwann cells containing myelin debris. In the early stages of remyelination the myelin sheath is very thin. Remyelinating segments at this time are easily detected amid a series of normally myelinated segments (*Figure 37*). As the myelin sheath becomes thicker and almost re-establishes its original adult thickness, the segments that were originally demyelinated can still be detected. Because three or four Schwann cells may be required to remyelinate each adult demyelinated segment (Fullerton *et al.*, 1965), sporadic series of short internodes 300–400 µm in length among normal internodes 1200 µm in length along the same fibre suggest previous segmental demyelination. If the segmental demyelination goes no further than nodal gap widening, remyelination may proceed by regrowth of the myelin back towards the node. When the nodal gap exceeds 15 µm, however, the deficiency in the sheath is usually repaired by a single Schwann cell which migrates in to form a short intercalated segment.

It is often difficult to estimate in teased preparations how many fibres within the whole nerve fascicle are involved in an acute demyelinating neuropathy. Transverse sections of epoxy resin-embedded nerve may be valuable in this respect. Much of the information may be gained from the examination of 1 µm sections stained with toluidine blue but electron microscopy is often valuable also. The main feature that will suggest segmental demyelination in these preparations is axon:myelin sheath disproportion (Weller and Das Gupta, 1968). In the early stages large axons devoid of myelin sheaths will be seen (*Figures 40* and *41*). Normally, non-myelinated nerves do not exceed 3 µm in

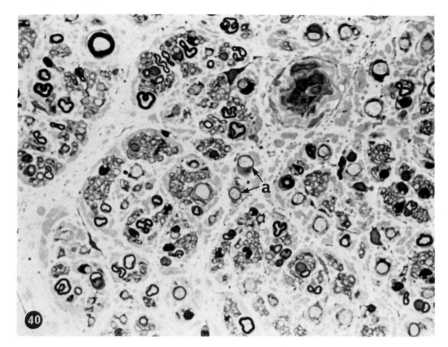

Fig. 40. Segmental demyelination: T.S. sural nerve showing many large axons (a) devoid of myelin sheaths. A normal myelinated fibre is seen top left. 1 µm Araldite section stained with toluidine blue. × 760

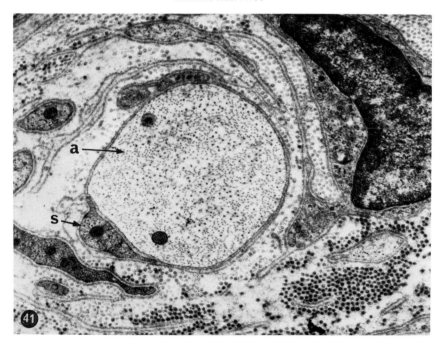

Fig. 41. Electron micrograph of a demyelinated 4 µm axon (a). Very little Schwann cytoplasm (s) is associated with the axon. × 15 200 (Courtesy of J. Neurol. Neurosurg. Psychiat.)

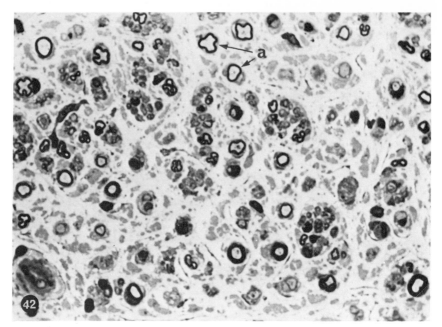

Fig. 42. Remyelination: T.S. sural nerve. Thinly myelinated remyelinated axons (a). Normally myelinated fibres are seen towards the bottom of the picture. 1 μm Araldite section stained with toluidine blue. × 760

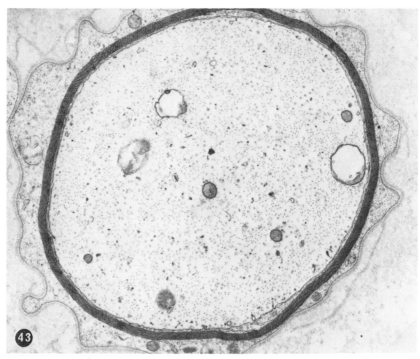

Fig. 43. Electron micrograph of a remyelinating axon with a disproportionately thin myelin sheath. × 20 600

diameter in man and most are between 0·5 and 2·0 μm (Ochoa and Mair, 1969a). There is very little overlap in size with myelinated axons, so if an axon is larger than 3 μm and lacks a myelin sheath, it is probably demyelinated. During the early stages of remyelination the myelin sheaths are disproportionately thin (*Figures 42* and *43*), but as they mature towards normal thickness, the remyelinated fibres may be difficult to differentiate from the unaffected fibres except, perhaps, for 'onion-bulb' whorl formation (Weller and Das Gupta, 1968) (see 'hypertrophic neuropathies' below).

Remyelinating fibres must be distinguished from swollen axon balloons seen during axon regeneration. The axon balloons are usually filled with mitochondria and other organelles; the myelin sheath is thin because it has been stretched to surround a greatly enlarged axon. Axons in the process of remyelination, on the other hand, are usually cytologically normal. Segmental demyelination can be detected in paraffin sections stained for axons (Palmgren or Bodian techniques) and for myelin (Luxol fast blue or Loyez) where there is loss of myelin but preservation of axons. Lymphocytic infiltration in allergic demyelination is also well demonstrated in paraffin sections. Lipid histochemical methods reveal myelin breakdown products and there is an increase in lysosomal enzyme staining.

NERVE CONDUCTION IN AXONAL DEGENERATION AND SEGMENTAL DEMYELINATION

Gilliatt and Hjorth (1972) divided the lateral popliteal nerve in the lower thigh in a series of baboons and studied the changes in nerve function and conduction that occurred in the distal part of the nerve. The muscle response to nerve stimulation disappeared after 4—5 days at a time when there was degeneration of nerve terminals. Conduction along the main portion of the nerve, however, was recordable for a further 2—3 days and there was little change in conduction velocity until the very late stages. During regeneration following axonal degeneration, conduction velocities are reduced, as fibres are small in diameter. When the nerve has fully regenerated, conduction velocities return to normal provided that enough large-diameter fibres recover.

Major changes in nerve conduction velocities occur in segmental demyelinating neuropathies (Thomas, 1971). In a normal myelinated nerve the impulse is conducted in a saltatory manner from node to node; when the myelin sheath is lost in segmental demyelination, conduction of the impulse is continuous and thus very much slower. Conduction velocities may be reduced by more than 50 per cent during the stages of demyelination and early remyelination in segmental demyelinating neuropathies.

HYPERTROPHIC NEUROPATHIES

Hypertrophic neuropathies form a group of chronic sensorimotor neuropathies characterized by thickening of peripheral nerve, segmental demyelination and the formation of 'onion-bulb' Schwann cell whorls within the nerve (*Figure 44*). In the later stages of the neuropathy there may be considerable loss of axons.

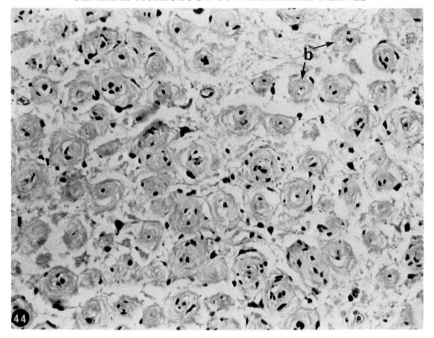

Fig. 44. T.S. nerve in hypertrophic neuropathy showing cellular 'onion-bulb' whorls (b) separated by endoneurial mucosubstance. H. and E. stain; × 300

Thickening of the nerve is due in part to the increased collagen content and cellularity of the nerve bundles; there is also often an increase in mucosubstance in the endoneurium. In severe cases the enlarged nerves are palpable through the skin and at biopsy they may appear grey and gelatinous macroscopically owing to the large amounts of endoneurial mucosubstance (Weller and Herzog, 1970).

Evidence of segmental demyelination and remyelination can be detected in teased fibres (Thomas and Lascelles, 1967) and in epoxy resin cross-sections of nerve by both light and electron microscopy (Weller, 1967). In the latter preparations large axons may be devoid of myelin, only thinly myelinated or in some cases possess a myelin sheath of normal thickness (Dyck *et al.*, 1968). The 'onion-bulb' whorls are best seen in transverse sections. They consist of imbricated layers of flat cell processes for the most part arranged around demyelinated or myelinated axons (Weller and Herzog, 1970). As the neuropathy progresses, axons degenerate and whorls are seen that are devoid of central axons. Most of the cell processes in the 'onion-bulb' whorls are Schwann cells (*Figure 45*); they are surrounded by basement membrane and some contain non-myelinated axons. The majority of non-myelinated axons are not involved in the whorls and form separate, distinct groups (Weller, 1967).

Bundles of collagen separate the cell layers in the whorl; the whorls are often separated by lakes of mucoid material *(Figure 44)* with histochemical staining characteristics of normal endoneurial mucosubstance (Weller and Das Gupta,

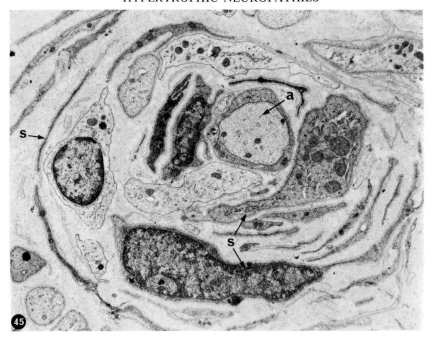

Fig. 45. Electron micrograph; T.S. of 'onion-bulb' whorl. The central demyelinated axon (a) is surrounded by a whorl of Schwann cells and their processes (s). × 7200 (Courtesy of Brain*)*

1968) containing fine fibrillary structures (Thomas and Lascelles, 1967).

'Onion-bulb' whorls are found in a wide variety of neuropathies (Pleasure and Towfighi, 1972) and the common factor appears to be segmental demyelination and remyelination, which in most cases is recurrent. Electron microscope studies have revealed that small 'onion-bulb' whorls form in many segmental demyelinating neuropathies (Weller and Das Gupta, 1968; Ballin and Thomas, 1969b; Dyck, 1969; Prineas and Wright, 1972). 'Onion-bulb' whorls do not form in nerves where there is repeated axonal degeneration and no segmental demyelination (Thomas, 1970).

The exact stimulus for formation of 'onion-bulb' whorls is not clear, nor is their function. Morris *et al.* (1972d) have described the separation of regenerating axons into compartments, and it has been suggested that the formation of 'onion-bulb' whorls is a similar attempt at compartmentalization in chronic segmental demyelinating neuropathies, possibly protecting the remyelinating fibres from disturbing factors in the endoneurium (Weller and Das Gupta, 1968; Morris *et al.*, 1972d). Clinically, hypertrophic neuropathies are usually chronic and progressive. The gross slowing of nerve conduction velocities reflects the widespread segmental demyelination in the affected nerves (Thomas and Lascelles, 1967). In the later stages there may be increasing axonal degeneration, with muscle wasting and contraction. Hypertrophic neuropathy should not be confused with other causes of thickened peripheral nerve, which include amyloidosis, leprosy and neurofibromatosis.

REFERENCES

Gombault and Mallet (1889) first described a sporadic case of hypertrophic neuropathy in 1889. A few years later Dejerine and Sottas (1893) reported a brother and sister with a severe type of hypertrophic neuropathy with a recessive pattern of inheritance (Dyck and Lambert, 1968). There is also a milder type of dominantly inherited hypertrophic neuropathy of Charcot–Marie–Tooth type, where the loss of large myelinated fibres and segmental demyelination may be a response to axonal atrophy (Dyck, Lais and Offord, 1974). Sporadic and familial cases of hypertrophic neuropathy have been reported in children (Weller, 1967; Lyon, 1969), where, despite the lack of myelin in the nerve, the children slowly develop. Rapidly progressive late-onset cases of hypertrophic neuropathy are often sporadic (Austin, 1956; Thomas and Lascelles, 1967; Weller, 1967). Pathological changes of hypertrophic neuropathy are characteristically found in Refsum's disease (Fardeau and Engel, 1969) and have been described in diabetic neuropathy (Ballin and Thomas, 1968) and various forms of polyneuropathy with segmental demyelination (Pleasure and Towfighi, 1972).

REFERENCES

Adams, C. W. M. (1965). In *Neurohistochemistry*. Amsterdam; Elsevier.
Adams, C. W. M. and Leibowitz, S. (1972). In *Research on Multiple Sclerosis*. Springfield, Illinois; Charles C. Thomas.
Aguayo, A. J., Martin, J. B. and Bray, G. M. (1972). 'Effects of nerve growth factor antiserum on peripheral unmyelinated nerve fibres.' *Acta Neuropath. (Berlin)*, **20**, 288.
Aguayo, A. J., Nair, C. P. V. and Bray, G. M. (1971). 'Peripheral nerve abnormalities in the Riley–Day syndrome.' *Arch. Neurol. (Chicago)*, **24**, 106.
Allt, G. (1969). 'Repair of segmental demyelination in peripheral nerves: an electron micoscope study.' *Brain*, **92**, 639.
Allt, G. and Cavanagh, J. B. (1969). 'Ultrastructural changes in the region of the node of Ranvier in the rat caused by diphtheria toxin.' *Brain*, **92**, 459.
Astrom, K.-E. and Waksman, B. H. (1962). 'The passive transfer of experimental allergic encephalomyelitis and neuritis with living lymphoid cells.' *J. Pathol. Bacteriol.*, **83**, 89.
Astrom, K. E., Webster, H. de F. and Arnason, B. G. (1968). 'The initial lesion in experimental allergic neuritis. A phase and electron microscope study.' *J. Exp. Med.*, **128**, 469.
Austin, J. H. (1956). 'Observations on the syndrome of hypertrophic neuritis (The hypertrophic interstitial radiculo-neuropathies).' *Medicine*, **35**, 187.
Ballin, R. H. M. and Thomas, P. K. (1968). 'Hypertrophic changes in diabetic neuropathy.' *Acta Neuropath. (Berlin)*, **11**, 93.
Ballin, R. H. M. and Thomas, P. K. (1969a). 'Electron microscope observations on demyelination and remyelination in experimental allergic neuritis. Part 1. Demyelination.' *J. Neurol. Sci.*, **8**, 1.
Ballin, R. H. M. and Thomas, P. K. (1969b). 'Electron microscope observations on demyelination and remyelination in experimental allergic neuritis. Part 2. Remyelination.' *J. Neurol. Sci.*, **8**, 225.
Ballin, R. H. M. and Thomas, P. K. (1969c). 'Changes at the node of Ranvier during Wallerian degeneration: an electron microscope study.' *Acta Neuropath. (Berlin)*, **14**, 237.
Bischoff, A., Fierz, U., Regli, F. and Ulrich, J. (1968). 'Peripherer-neurologische Störungen bei der Fabryschen Krankheit (Angiokeratoma corporis diffusum universale) klinisch-elektronen mikroskopische Befunde bei Fall.' *Klin. Wschr.*, **46**, 666.
Blinzinger, K. and Kreutzberg, G. (1968). 'Displacement of synaptic terminals from regenerating motor neurones by microglial cells.' *Z. Zellforsch.*, **85**, 145.
Bradley, W. G. (1974). 'The neuropathies.' In *Disorders of Voluntary Muscle*, p. 804. Ed. by J. N. Walton. Edinburgh; Churchill Livingstone.
Bradley, W. G. and Asbury, A. K. (1970). 'The duration of synthesis phase in neurilemma cells in the mouse sciatic nerve during degeneration.' *Exp. Neurol.*, **26**, 275.

REFERENCES

Bradley, W. G. and Jennekens, F. G. I. (1971). 'Axonal degeneration in dipththeritic neuropathy.' *J. Neurol. Sci.*, **13**, 415.

Bradley, W. G. and Williams, M. H. (1973). 'Axoplasmic flow in axonal neuropathies. I. Axoplasmic flow in cats with toxic neuropathies.' *Brain*, **96**, 235.

Brain, W. R. and Walton, J. N. (1969). In *Brain's Diseases of the Nervous System*, 7th edn. London; Oxford University Press.

Brownell, B., Oppenheimer, D. R. and Spalding, J. M. K. (1972). 'Neurogenic muscle atrophy in myasthenia gravis.' *J. Neurol. Neurosurg. Psychiat.*, **35**, 311.

Cajal, S. R. y (1928). In *Degeneration and Regeneration of the Nervous System*. London; Oxford University Press.

Cavanagh, J. B. (1964). 'The significance of the dying-back process in experimental and human neurological disease.' *Int. Rev. exp. Pathol.*, **7**, 219.

Cavanagh, J. B. (1973). 'Peripheral neuropathy caused by chemical agents'. *CRC Critical Reviews in Toxicology*, November 1973, p.365.

Cavanagh, J. B. and Chen, F. C. K. (1971). 'Amino acid incorporation into protein during the "silent phase" before organo-mercury and pBPAU neuropathy in the rat.' *Acta Neuropath. (Berlin)*, **19**, 216.

Cavanagh, J. B. and Jacobs, J. (1964). 'Some quantitative aspects of diphtheritic neuropathy.' *Br. J. Exp. Pathol.*, **45**, 309.

Cavanagh, J. B., Passingham, R. J. and Vogt, J. A. (1964). 'Staining of sensory and motor nerves in muscles with Sudan black B.' *J. Pathol. Bacteriol.*, **88**, 89.

Cervós-Navarro, J. (1962). 'Elektronenmikroskopische Untersuchungen an retrograd Veränderten Spinalganglien.' *Fortschr. Med.*, **80**, 751.

Cragg, B. G. and Thomas, P. K. (1964). 'The conduction velocity of regenerated peripheral nerve fibres.' *J. Physiol. (London)*, **171**, 164.

Dayan, A. D., Ogul, E. and Graveson, G. S. (1972). 'Polyneuritis and herpes zoster.' *J. Neurol. Neurosurg. Psychiat.*, **35**, 170.

Dejerine, J. and Sottas, J. (1893). 'Sur la névrite interstitielle, hypertrophique et progressive de l'enfance.' *Compt. Rend. Soc. Biol.*, **45**, 63.

Dubowitz, V. and Brooke, M.H. (1973). In *Muscle Biopsy: A Modern Approach*. London; Saunders.

Duchen, L. W. (1971). 'An electron microscope study of the changes induced by Botulinum toxin in the motor end-plates of slow and fast muscle fibres of the mouse.' *J. Neurol. Sci.*, **14**, 47.

Dyck, P. J., Conn, D. L. and Okazaki, H. (1972). 'Necrotizing angiopathic neuropathy. Three-dimensional morphology of fiber degeneration related to sites of occluded vessels.' *Mayo Clin. Proc.*, **47**, 461.

Dyck, P. J. and Gomez, M. R. (1968). 'Segmental demyelinisation in Dejerine–Sottas disease.' *Mayo Clin. Proc.*, **43**, 280.

Dyck, P. J., Gutrecht, J. A., Bastron, J. A., Karnes, W. E. and Dale, A. J. D. (1968). 'Histologic and teased-fiber measurements of sural nerve in disorders of lower motor and primary sensory neurones.' *Mayo Clin. Proc.*, **43**, 81.

Dyck, P. J. and Hopkins, A. P. (1972). 'Electron microscopic observations on degeneration and regeneration of unmyelinated fibres.' *Brain*, **95**, 223.

Dyck, P. J., Lais, A. C. and Offord, K. P. (1974). 'The nature of myelinated nerve fibre degeneration in dominantly inherited hypertrophic neuropathy.' *Mayo Clin. Proc.*, **49**, 34.

Dyck, P. J. and Lambert, E. H. (1968). 'Lower motor and primary sensory neuron diseases with peroneal muscular atrophy. I. Neurologic, genetic and electrophysiologic findings in hereditary polyneuropathies.' *Arch. Neurol.*, **18**, 603.

Dyck, P. J. and Lambert, E. H. (1969). 'Dissociated sensation in amyloidosis: compound action potential; quantitative histologic and teased-fiber, and electron microscopic studies of sural nerve biopsies.' *Arch. Neurol.*, **20**, 490.

Eames, R. A. and Lange, L. S. (1967). 'Clinical and pathological study of ischaemic neuropathy.' *J. Neurol. Neurosurg. Psychiat.*, **20**, 215.

Fardeau, M. and Engel, W. K. (1969). 'Ultrastructural study of a peripheral nerve biopsy in Refsum's disease.' *J. Neuropath. Exp. Neurol.*, **28**, 278.

Fisher, C. M. and Adams, R. D. (1956). 'Diphtheritic paralysis: a pathological study.' *J. Neuropath. Exp. Neurol.*, **15**, 243.

Fullerton, P. M. (1966). 'Chronic peripheral neuropathy produced by lead poisoning in guinea pigs.' *J. Neuropath. Exp. Neurol.*, **25**, 214.

REFERENCES

Fullerton, P. M. and Barnes, J. M. (1966). 'Peripheral neuropathy in rats produced by acrylamide.' *Br. J. Indust. Med.,* **23,** 210.

Fullerton, P. M., Gilliatt, R. W., Lascelles, R. G. and Morgan-Hughes, J. A. (1965). 'Relation between fibre diameter and internodal length in chronic neuropathy.' *J. Physiol (London),* **178,** 26P.

Gilliatt, R. W. and Hjorth, R. J. (1972). 'Nerve conduction during Wallerian degeneration in the baboon.' *J. Neurol. Neurosurg. Psychiat.,* **35,** 335.

Gombault, A. (1880). 'Contribution à l'étude anatomique de la névrite parenchymateuse subaiguë et chronique—Névrite segmentaire péri-axile.' *Arch. Neurol. (Paris),* **1,** 11.

Gombault, A. and Mallet, (1889). 'Un cas de tabès ayant débuté dans l'enfance: autopsie.' *Arch. Med. Exp.,* **1,** 385.

Hallpike, J. F. (1972). 'Enzyme and protein changes in myelin breakdown and multiple sclerosis.' *Progr. Histochem. Cytochem.,* **3,** 179.

Holtzman, E. and Novikoff, A. B. (1965). 'Lysosomes in the rat sciatic nerve following crush.' *J. Cell Biol.,* **27,** 651.

Hopkins, A. P. and Lambert, E. H. (1972). 'Conduction in regenerating unmyelinated fibres.' *Brain,* **95,** 213.

Hughes, J. T. (1966). In *Pathology of the Spinal Cord.* London; Lloyd-Luke.

Jacobs, J. M., Cavanagh, J. B. and Mellick, R. S. (1966). 'Intraneural injection of diphtheria toxin.' *Br. J. Exp. Pathol.,* **47,** 507.

Knowles, M., Hughes, D., Caspary, E. A. and Field, E. J. (1968). 'Lymphocyte transformation in the Guillain–Barré syndrome.' *Lancet,* **ii,** 1207.

Kreutzberg, G. W. (1972). 'Neural degeneration and regeneration.' In *Pathology of the Nervous System,* Vol. III, p. 2678. Ed. by J. Minckler. New York; McGraw-Hill.

Kreutzberg, G. W. and Schubert, P. (1971). 'Changes in axonal flow during regeneration of mammalian motor nerves.' *Acta Neuropath., Suppl.,* **5,** 70.

Lampert, P. W. and Schochet, S. S. (1968). 'Demyelination and remyelination in lead neuropathy. Electron microscope studies.' *J. Neuropath. Exp. Neurol.,* **27,** 527.

Leibowitz, S. (1972). In *Research on Multiple Sclerosis,* by C. W. M. Adams and S. Leibowitz. Springfield, Illinois; Charles C. Thomas.

Liversedge, L. A. and Campbell, M. J. (1974). 'The central neuronal muscular atrophies and other dysfunctions of the anterior horn cells.' In *Disorders of Voluntary Muscle,* p. 775. Ed. by J. N. Walton. Edinburgh; Churchill Livingstone.

Lyon, G. (1969). 'Ultrastructural study of a nerve biopsy from a case of early infantile chronic neuropathy.' *Acta Neuropath.,* **13,** 131.

Morgan-Hughes, J. A. and Engel, W. K. (1968). 'Structural and histochemical changes in the axons following nerve crush.' *Arch. Neurol.,* **19,** 598.

Morris, J. H., Hudson, A. R. and Weddell, G. (1972a). 'A study of degeneration and regeneration in the divided rat sciatic nerve. I. The traumatic degeneration of myelin in the proximal stump of the divided nerve.' *Z. Zellforsch.,* **124,** 76.

Morris, J. H., Hudson, A. R. and Weddell, G. (1972b). 'A study of degeneration and regeneration in the divided rat sciatic nerve. II. The development of the regenerating unit.' *Z. Zellforsch.,* **124,** 103.

Morris, J. H., Hudson, A. R. and Weddell, G. (1972c). 'A study of degeneration and regeneration in the divided rat sciatic nerve. III. Changes in the axons of the proximal stump.' *Z. Zellforsch.,* **124,** 131.

Morris, J. H., Hudson, A. R. and Weddell, G. (1972d). 'A study of degeneration and regeneration in the divided rat sciatic nerve. IV. Changes in fascicular microtopography perineurium and endoneurial fibroblasts.' *Z. Zellforsch.,* **124,** 165.

Nathaniel, E. J. H. and Pease, D. C. (1963a). 'Degenerative changes in rat dorsal roots during Wallerian degeneration.' *J. Ultrastruct. Res.,* **9,** 511.

Nathaniel, E. J. H. and Pease, D. C. (1963b). 'Regenerative changes in rat dorsal root following Wallerian degeneration.' *J. Ultrastruct. Res.,* **9,** 533.

Ochoa, J. and Mair, W. G. P. (1969a). 'The normal sural nerve in man. I. Ultrastructure and numbers of fibres and cells.' *Acta. Neuropath. (Berlin),* **13,** 197.

Ochoa, J. and Mair, W. G. P. (1969b). 'The normal sural nerve in man. II. Changes in the axons and Schwann cells due to ageing.' *Acta Neuropath. (Berlin),* **13,** 217.

Pleasure, D. E., Feldman, B. and Prockop, D. J. (1973). 'Diphtheria toxin inhibits the synthesis of myelin proteolipid and basic proteins by peripheral nerve *in vitro.' J. Neurochem.,* **20,** 81.

Pleasure, D. E. and Towfighi, J. (1972). 'Onion-bulb neuropathies.' *Arch Neurol.,* **26,** 289.

Prineas, J. (1969a). 'The pathogenesis of dying-back neuropathies. Part 1: An ultrastructural

REFERENCES

study of experimental triorthocresyl phosphate poisoning.' *J. Neuropath. Exp. Neurol.,* **28,** 571.

Prineas, J. (1969b). 'The pathogenesis of dying-back neuropathies. Part 2: An ultrastructural study of experimental acrylamide intoxication in the rat.' *J. Neuropath. Exp. Neurol.,* **28,** 598.

Prineas, J. W. (1972). 'Acute idiopathic polyneuritis: an electron microscope study.' *Lab. Invest.,* **26,** 133.

Prineas, J. W. and Wright, R. G. (1972). 'The fine structure of peripheral nerve lesions in a virus-induced demyelinating disease in fowl (Marek's disease).' *Lab. Invest.,* **26,** 548.

Schröder, J. M. (1968). 'Die Hyperneurotisation Büngnerscher Bänder bei der experimentellen Isoniazid-Neuropathie: phasenkontrast und electronmikroskopische Untersuchungen.' *Virchows Arch. Zellpath. Abt. B,* **1,** 131.

Thomas, P. K. (1970). 'The cellular response to nerve injury. 3. The effect of repeated crush injuries.' *J. Anat.,* **106,** 463.

Thomas, P. K. (1971). 'The morphological basis for alterations in nerve conduction in peripheral neuropathy.' *Proc. Roy. Soc. Med.,* **64,** 295.

Thomas, P. K. (1973). 'The ultrastructural pathology of unmyelinated nerve fibres.' In *New Developments in Electromyography and Clinical Neurophysiology,* Vol. 2, p. 227. Ed. by J. E. Desmedt. Basle; Karger.

Thomas, P. K., King, R. H. M. and Phelps, A. C. (1972). 'Electron microscope observations on the degeneration of unmyelinated fibres following nerve section.' *J. Anat.,* **113,** 279.

Thomas, P. K. and Lascelles, R. G. (1967). 'Hypertrophic neuropathy.' *Quart. J. Med.,* **36,** 223.

Waksman, B. H. and Adams, R. D. (1955). 'Allergic neuritis: an experimental disease of rabbits induced by the injection of peripheral nervous tissue and adjuvants.' *J. Exp. Med.,* **102,** 213.

Waller, A. (1850). 'Experiments on the section of the glossopharyngeal and hypoglossal nerves of the frog and observations of the alterations produced thereby in the structure of their primitive fibres.' *Phil. Trans. Roy. Soc.,* **140,** 423.

Weller, R. O. (1965). 'Diphtheritic neuropathy in the chicken: an electron microscope study.' *J. Pathol. Bacteriol.,* **89,** 591.

Weller, R. O. (1967). 'An electron microscope study of hypertrophic neuropathy of Dejerine–Sottas.' *J. Neurol. Neurosurg. Psychiat.,* **30,** 111.

Weller, R. O., Bruckner, F. E. and Chamberlain, M. A. (1970). 'Rheumatoid neuropathy: a histological and electrophysiological study.' *J. Neurol. Neurosurg. Psychiat.,* **33,** 592.

Weller, R. O. and Das Gupta, T. K. (1968). 'Experimental hypertrophic neuropathy: an electron microscope study.' *J. Neurol. Neurosurg. Psychiat.,* **31,** 34.

Weller, R. O. and Herzog, I. (1970). 'Schwann cell lysosomes in hypertrophic neuropathy and in normal human nerves.' *Brain,* **93,** 347.

Weller, R. O. and Mellick, R. S. (1966). 'Acid phosphatase and lysosome activity in diphtheritic neuropathy and Wallerian degeneration'. *Br. J. Exp. Pathol.,* **47,** 426.

Weller, R. O. and Nester, B. (1972). 'Early changes at the node of Ranvier in segmental demyelination: histochemical and electron microscopic observations.' *Brain,* **95,** 665.

Williams, P. L. and Hall, S. M. (1971). 'Prolonged *in vivo* observations of normal peripheral nerve fibres and their acute reactions to crush and deliberate trauma.' *J. Anat.,* **108,** 379.

Wisniewski, H., Prineas, J. and Raine, C. S. (1969). 'An ultrastructural study of experimental demyelination and remyelination. I. Acute experimental allergic encephalomyelitis in the peripheral nervous system.' *Lab. Invest.,* **21,** 105.

5

Pathology of Peripheral Nerve Diseases

INTRODUCTION

In many cases the interpretation of pathological features in peripheral nerves is difficult without adequate clinical data. It is important therefore that these data should be available to the pathologist before the specimen of nerve is taken. This is especially true if a nerve biopsy is to be performed, as the small amount of tissue available must be suitably apportioned for the more informative technical procedures. For example, if metachromatic leukodystrophy is suspected, lipid histochemical or biochemical studies for the detection of sulphatide are very important, so the tissue should not all be embedded in paraffin or epoxy resin, as the diagnosis may be difficult to establish from this material.

A short account of the clinical features and investigation of peripheral neuropathies is given in this chapter. More detailed accounts will be found in standard textbooks of clinical neurology (Brain and Walton, 1969; Vinken and Bruyn, 1970; Bradley, 1975).

CLINICAL FEATURES OF PERIPHERAL NEUROPATHIES

The clinical features of a peripheral neuropathy depend upon the distribution and severity of the nerve damage and upon whether the disease process affects motor or sensory nerves or both.

Sensory symptoms may present as loss of certain sensations. When large-diameter myelinated fibres in the nerve are affected, the patient complains of numbness; touch sensation and joint position sense may be impaired, so that the patient may be ataxic and unable to identify objects in the dark. Loss of impairment of function in the small myelinated and non-myelinated fibres in the nerve results in loss of pain and temperature sensation; this may be accompanied by ulcer formation in repeatedly injured, insensitive parts of the body. In addition to the loss of sensation, distressing, abnormal sensations may occur. Nerve compression frequently results in pain, whereas non-compressive neuropathies are often marked by paraesthesiae, lightning pains and burning sensations; light touch and pin-prick may be very painful. These abnormal sensations may be due to the aberrant patterns of input into the nervous system that result from damage to selected nerve fibres.

Motor symptoms usually present as weakness and rapid fatigue of muscle groups supplied by the affected nerves. If there is a significant degree of axon degeneration involving motor nerve fibres, fibrillation and muscle wasting may be seen.

Tendon reflexes are lost very early in peripheral neuropathies where there is damage to the sensory or motor fibres supplying the muscle spindles, or to the motor nerves supplying extrafusal muscle fibres.

Involvement of the autonomic nervous system in diseases that affect the spinal cord, sympathetic chain and ganglia, or the autonomic nerves themselves, produces a variety of visceral symptoms and signs. These include orthostatic hypotension, impotence, vasodilatation in the skin and bladder atonia.

CLINICAL CLASSIFICATION OF PERIPHERAL NEUROPATHIES

As the aetiology of many peripheral neuropathies is, at present, unknown, one very useful approach to their classification is through their patterns of clinical presentation. Most common is the type of neuropathy which presents as a mixed sensorimotor distal symmetrical neuropathy with a glove and stocking loss of sensation and weakness of the distal limb muscles producing foot drop and weakness of the small muscles of the hand. Some patients have a distal symmetrical neuropathy which is purely sensory or purely motor. A less frequent presentation occurs when just one nerve is involved, as in trauma and in some vascular neuropathies. If several individual nerves are involved, it is called a mononeuritis multiplex; this can usually be distinguished from a polyneuropathy by its asymmetrical distribution. The most frequent cause of mononeuritis multiplex is vascular disease. The term 'neuritis' now appears to be used interchangeably with the more common term 'neuropathy' and not just for inflammatory diseases of peripheral nerves. A proximal motor neuropathy is sometimes seen. Pure autonomic neuropathies are rare but they may be expressed as part of a sensorimotor polyneuropathy.

The time course and progression of neuropathies varies. Acute peripheral neuropathies develop within 3 weeks, whereas subacute neuropathies take a little longer, 3–12 weeks. Such neuropathies may resolve, remain stationary or relapse. Most common are the chronic, progressive unremitting neuropathies, where the development of signs and symptoms spans more than 3 months.

CLINICAL INVESTIGATION OF PERIPHERAL NEUROPATHIES

In addition to the clinical history, family history and physical examination of the patient, there are a number of clinical investigations which may be valuable in determining the cause of the peripheral neuropathy. Ideally, these investigations should be completed before a peripheral nerve biopsy is performed, so that the maximum amount of information is available to the pathologist when he examines the nerve.

The type of clinical investigation undertaken will be determined by the clinical history and physical findings. Radiographic examination of the spine for intervertebral disc lesions or neoplastic lesions will be important in the investigation of isolated root lesions. Other entrapment neuropathies may accompany bony or joint abnormalities, as in rheumatoid arthritis. Haematological investigations and serum biochemistry may reveal vitamin deficiencies (e.g. B_{12}) or abnormal levels of lead, glucose, phytanic acid, etc. Examination of the urine for sulphatide granules or arylsulphatase A activity is an important investigation for metachromatic leukodystrophy. The cytology and protein levels in cerebrospinal fluid often add useful information. Creatine phosphokinase levels in the serum are usually normal in neuropathies except where there is acute, widespread denervation; a raised blood level of this enzyme most frequently suggests primary muscle disease.

Electrophysiological studies are a very important part of the investigation of a patient with a peripheral neuropathy. Electromyography and measurements of nerve conduction are used extensively to distinguish between peripheral nerve disease and primary muscle disease. It is also possible, by these techniques, to determine whether a neuropathy is due mainly to axonal degeneration or segmental demyelination.

Electromyography (EMG)

In clinical electromyography recordings are made with a concentric needle electrode, 0·5 mm in diameter, inserted into the muscle. The needle has a bevelled tip and the central core is insulated from the outer casing; potential differences between the inner and outer parts of the electrode are amplified and displayed on an oscilloscope or monitored on a speaker (Calne and Pallis, 1972).

Normal muscle

A characteristic recording is obtained when an electromyography needle is inserted into a normal muscle; the record is altered in a denervated or myopathic muscle. In a normal muscle many fibres are innervated by the terminal arborization of a single motor nerve axon; this group of muscle fibres is termed a motor unit (Buchthal and Rosenfalck, 1973). When a single motor nerve fibre is stimulated, the electrical recording (action potential) from its motor unit has a characteristic diphasic or triphasic wave-form. The amplitude of this wave-form depends upon the number of muscle fibres in the unit, whereas the duration of the wave-form is a reflection of the area over which the muscle fibres in the motor unit are distributed. With the onset of voluntary muscular contraction, more units are recruited and recordings from single motor units become overshadowed by the electrical activity from neighbouring motor units. This is called the interference or recruitment pattern.

Denervation

Fairly specific electromyographic changes are seen in muscles where denervation has occurred due either to loss of lower motor neurones or to axonal degeneration in peripheral nerves. These changes fall into four main categories: fibrillation, fasciculation, giant motor unit potentials and reduction in the interference or recruitment pattern.

Fibrillation potentials are small spontaneous discharges from single muscle fibres or groups of fibres that can be recorded some 2 weeks after denervation; they persist until the muscle is very atrophic. Fasciculation is spontaneous activity of greater amplitude involving whole motor units and, unlike fibrillation, may be clinically visible. The wave-forms are frequently bizarre and irregular, occurring most often in chronic lesions of anterior horn cells, such as motor neurone disease. Giant motor unit potentials are characteristic of chronic neuropathies, poliomyelitis and motor neurone disease, where there is incomplete denervation; the surviving axons form sprouts which re-innervate neighbouring denervated muscle fibres, and this leads to enlargement of the motor units. The reduction in the number of motor units in a denervated muscle diminishes the interference or recruitment pattern on voluntary muscle activity.

Primary muscle disease

One of the characteristics of many myopathies and dystrophies is the loss of individual muscle fibres. This results in a reduction of the number of fibres in the motor units, so that the action potential is low in amplitude and of brief duration. Furthermore, the smooth diphasic or triphasic wave-form of the normal EMG is broken up into a polyphasic pattern with multiple spikes. If there is patchy inflammation within the muscle, some features of denervation may be seen in addition to the characteristic myopathic pattern; the denervation is probably a result of separation of the muscle fibres from their nerve supply by the inflammatory lesions. In myotonic disorders the muscle fibres are very sensitive to mechanical stimuli and insertion of the needle electrode induces high frequency repetitive discharges; the noise of this abnormal activity on the audio-monitor has been likened to a dive-bomber.

Quantitative techniques and computer analyses are being increasingly used to examine polyphasic activity in EMG and to provide a measure of abnormality in primary muscle disorders and to distinguish them from neurogenic lesions (Hayward and Willison, 1973; Lee and White, 1973).

Nerve conduction studies

Motor nerve conduction velocities can be calculated by measuring the time intervals between stimulating the nerve, at a specified distance proximal to a muscle, and the response in the muscle. The nerves most commonly used in routine examinations are the median nerve in the forearm (recording from abductor pollicis brevis muscle in the hand) and the common peroneal nerve in the leg (recording from extensor digitorum brevis (e.d.b.) in the foot). A needle electrode is inserted into the e.d.b. muscle, for example, and the common peroneal nerve is stimulated electrically, both at the knee and at the instep (anterior tibial nerve).

The time interval between the initial stimulus and the response in the muscle is the latency. If the terminal latency of the response (elicited by stimulating at the instep) is subtracted from the total latency (evoked by stimulating at the knee), a figure is obtained which represents the time taken for the impulse to travel from knee to instep. This distance is measured with a tape-measure and the conduction velocity along the nerve is calculated in metres per second (normal range 40–60 m s^{-1}). Conduction velocities in the median and ulnar nerves can be measured in a similar way (normal range, 50–70 m s^{-1}).

Direct recordings of action potentials from superficial nerves can be made through the skin, or from needle recording electrodes inserted near the nerve. Thus, the anterior tibial nerve can be stimulated at the instep and the action potential recorded at the knee. This technique is particularly valuable for measuring conduction in sensory nerves. If a stimulating ring electrode is placed on the index finger, the action potential can be recorded over the median nerve at the wrist. Similarly, the ulnar nerve is stimulated by an electrode on the little finger and recordings are made at the elbow. Clinical techniques for measuring nerve conduction velocity *in vivo* relate only to the large-diameter fibres; however, conduction velocities of small myelinated fibres and non-myelinated axons can be measured *in vitro* by studying the evoked potentials in a length of nerve taken at biopsy (Lambert and Dyck, 1968).

Disorders of nerve conduction

Nerve conduction studies are invaluable for distinguishing neuropathies that are due to axonal degeneration from those that are due mainly to segmental demyelination (Gilliatt, 1973). Conduction along a degenerating axon continues for a few days after the injury and then stops, with very little slowing of conduction; it is an 'all or none' phenomenon. In neuropathies where there is extensive axonal degeneration the conduction velocity may be reduced by a small amount owing to the loss of large-diameter fast-conducting fibres; decrease in the amplitude of the action potential in such a nerve reflects the overall loss of fibres. In 'dying back' neuropathies the distal latency is increased owing to the degeneration of the distal end of the motor nerves. During the early stages of axonal regeneration conduction velocities are very slow and usually only return to 60–75 per cent of normal values after 2–3 years (Gilliatt, 1973). Localized slowing of nerve conduction may occur at sites of nerve compression in entrapment neuropathies. However, the most marked reduction in nerve conduction velocity is seen in segmental demyelinating neuropathies, e.g. Guillain–Barré syndrome, diphtheria, diabetes and hypertrophic neuropathy, where the nerve conduction may be slowed by 30 per cent or more.

Electromyography and nerve conduction studies may give useful information about spinal root lesions. Segmental demyelination may be confined to the roots, and in these cases there may be no detectable abnormality in the more peripheral parts of the nerve despite the clinical signs of nerve dysfunction. Axonal degeneration in the anterior, motor roots may be deduced from patterns of denervation in the muscles supplied by the affected segments. In sensory roots nerve damage, lesions can occur either central to the dorsal root ganglion or peripheral to it. If there is degeneration of the central axons bound for the posterior columns of the spinal cord, the peripheral parts of the sensory nerve will remain intact. However, if the link with the central nervous system is broken, the symptoms will persist, as there is little chance of regeneration. When the nerve distal to the ganglion is damaged, axonal degeneration may be detected in the more peripheral part of the sensory nerve.

Disorders of neuromuscular transmission occur mainly in myasthenia gravis and the Eaton–Lambert (myasthenic) syndrome. In myasthenia gravis repeated rapid nerve stimulation leads to a progressive decrease in the amplitude of muscle action potentials, whereas in the Eaton–Lambert syndrome similar stimulation produces an increase in the amplitude of the muscle action potential.

Incidence of peripheral neuropathies

The three major causes of peripheral neuropathies throughout the world are leprosy, diabetes and old age (Bradley, 1974). A fourth group of 'undiagnosed' chronic progressive sensorimotor distal neuropathies may account for 40 per cent of the peripheral neuropathies in Britain (Prineas, 1970). In an industrialized society the total incidence of peripheral neuropathies is at least 50 per 100 000 per year (Bradley, 1974). A local survey in Carlisle (Brewis *et al.*, 1966) revealed an incidence of 2·3 per 100 000 per year for carpal tunnel syndrome, 0·6 per 100 000 per year for Guillain–Barré syndrome and 0·2 per 100 000 per year for peroneal muscular atrophy.

PATHOLOGY OF PERIPHERAL
NERVE DISEASES

Disease processes may affect peripheral nerves at any point from the anterior horn cell or sensory ganglion to the neuro-muscular junction or sensory ending. The classification of peripheral nerve pathology employed here is based upon several factors, but chiefly upon the anatomical site of the lesion, the aetiology of the disease and its histopathology. Most emphasis has been given to the peripheral nerve diseases where there is a definite histopathological basis; a more extensive and detailed classification has been published by the Research Group on Neuromuscular Diseases (Walton, 1968).

CLASSIFICATION OF PERIPHERAL NERVE
DISEASES

1. Disorders of the Vertebral Column and Spinal Cord

    (a) Developmental disorders (myelodysplasia): spina bifida, myelomeningocele.

(b) Trauma and compression of the spinal cord and nerve roots. Penetrating wounds, fractures, spondylosis, disc protrusions, metabolic bone disease, metastatic and primary tumours.

(c) Infections: osteomyelitis, meningitis, myelitis.

(d) Syringomyelia.

(e) Vascular disorders.

(f) Multiple sclerosis.

(g) Motor neurone disease.

(h) Spinal muscular atrophies: Werdnig–Hoffman disease; Kugelberg–Welander disease; arthrogryposis.

2. Hereditary Peripheral Neuropathies

(a) Peroneal muscular atrophy and hypertrophic neuropathy:
  (i) Charcot–Marie–Tooth disease with hypertrophic neuropathy and dominant inheritance.
  (ii) Dejerine–Sottas disease with hypertrophic neuropathy and recessive inheritance.
  (iii) Neuronal type of Charcot–Marie–Tooth disease with dominant inheritance.
  (iv) Charcot–Marie–Tooth disease with progressive spinal muscular atrophy.
  (v) Infantile hypertrophic neuropathy.

(b) Friedreich's ataxia.

(c) Hereditary sensory neuropathy:
  (i) Dominant.
  (ii) Recessive.
  (iii) Familial dysautonomia (Riley–Day syndrome).

(d) Peripheral neuropathies in disorders of lipid metabolism:
  (i) Metachromatic leukodystrophy (sulphatide lipidosis).
  (ii) Krabbe's globoid cell leukodystrophy.
  (iii) Fabry's disease.
  (iv) Refsum's disease.
  (v) Disorders of lipoprotein metabolism.

(e) Amyloidosis—primary, B-lymphocyte dyscrasias, secondary. Familial amyloidosis.
  (i) Portuguese familial amyloidosis (Andrade type).
  (ii) Indiana–Maryland familial amyloidosis (Rukavina type).
  (iii) Iowa familial amyloidosis (van Allen type).

(f) Acute intermittent porphyria.

3. Traumatic Nerve Lesions.

4. Entrapment and Compression Neuropathies.

5. Neuropathies due to Vascular Disease: Atherosclerosis, arteritis, rheumatoid neuropathy.

6. Neuropathies due to Toxic Substances.

7. Metabolic Neuropathies:
  (a) Diabetic neuropathy.
  (b) Neuropathies due to vitamin deficiencies.

(c) Uraemic neuropathy.
(d) Endocrine disorders.
(e) Amyloidosis (see 2e).

8. Inflammatory Disorders of Peripheral Nerves:
    (a) Guillain–Barré syndrome (acute post-infective polyneuritis).
    (b) Virus infections: poliomyelitis, herpes zoster (varicella zoster).
    (c) Leprosy.

9. Neuropathy in Malignant Disease:
    (a) Metastatic involvement.
    (b) Non-metastatic (remote) effects of malignant disease.

10. Peripheral Neuropathies in the Aged.

11. Autonomic Neuropathies.

12. Myasthenia gravis.

DISORDERS OF THE VERTEBRAL COLUMN AND SPINAL CORD

Developmental disorders (Myelodysplasia)

Defects in neural tube development vary in their severity. Spina bifida occulta is a mild form in which there is failure of fusion of the vertebral laminae. This is most common at the lumbosacral level, and although the cord may not be directly affected, there are often fibrous adhesions in the leptomeningeal covering of the cord and damage to the spinal nerve roots may ensue (James and Lassman, 1967). In anterior spina bifida the vertebral bodies are split (Hughes, 1966); more extensive disorders may be found with connections between the gut and neural tube (Willis, 1962).

Meningocele or myelomeningocele often complicates spina bifida. A sac containing cerebrospinal fluid (CSF) protrudes posteriorly from the spinal canal, usually in the lumbar region. The wall of the sac consists of dermal elements and adherent dura (meningocele) and frequently the flattened, disorganized spinal cord and nerve roots adhere to the sac wall (myelomeningocele). Early closure of the sac may prevent the infection which often spreads to involve the ventricles in the brain. Tissue taken from the wall of the sac often contains islands of glial tissue, neurones and nerve roots embedded in the subcutaneous or dermal regions. The nervous tissue in these specimens is most easily detected in paraffin sections with haematoxylin van Gieson stain; the pale yellow stained central nervous elements contrast with the red collagenous dermal tissue.

Hydrocephalus is a common complication in babies with myelomeningocele due to the presence of an associated Arnold–Chiari malformation of the lower brain stem and cerebellum (Milhorat, 1972). There is also a variable degree of motor and sensory deficit affecting the lower limbs and bladder due to involvement of the spinal cord and nerve roots in the myelomeningocele sac. Peripheral nerves in the legs show reduction of axons and the muscles undergo denervation atrophy.

Early antepartum diagnosis of some neural tube abnormalities, including anencephaly and myelodysplasias, is now possible if there is a high level of α-fetoprotein in the amniotic fluid (Stewart and Ward, 1974).

Trauma and compression of spinal cord and nerve roots

Penetrating wounds, fractures and haemorrhage into the spinal cord will not only damage the ascending and descending tracts of the cord, but also destroy motor neurones in the anterior horns of grey matter and nerve roots at the site of the injury. Compression of the cord and nerve roots occurs in cervical spondylosis and in intervertebral disc protrusion (Hughes, 1966). Spondylotic protrusions into the lateral part of the spinal canal or into the intervertebral foramina most frequently compress the posterior (sensory) roots and cause pain in the areas they supply. The anterior roots are frequently spared, but if they are compressed, there is weakness and wasting of the muscles supplied by the affected segments. The pathology of the acute lesions in the roots is probably similar to that seen in peripheral nerves at other sites of compression (Neary and Eames, 1975), i.e. oedema of the nerve, segmental demyelination and axonal degeneration. Spinal cord and nerve root compression may be a complication of vertebral collapse in metabolic bone disease, deposition of metastatic tumour or the growth of primary tumours, e.g. ependymoma, meningioma, within the spinal canal.

Infections

Pyogenic osteomyelitis or tuberculosis of the vertebral column may result in cord or spinal root compression. Chronic arachnoiditis with fibrous adhesions involving the spinal nerves may follow leptomeningitis. Syphilitic infections cause a lepto- and pachymeningitis with an arteritis and gummata in the meninges. The primary lesion in the dorsal roots in tabes dorsalis is probably due to fibrous thickening and chronic inflammation in the leptomeninges covering the dorsal roots and posterior aspects of the cord (Hughes, 1966). Lymphocyte and plasma cell infiltration is seen in the meninges in tabes with axonal degeneration and gliosis of the posterior columns of the spinal cord, especially in the lower thoracic and lumbar regions. The sensory fibres in peripheral nerves are not usually affected.

Infection of the central nervous system with poliomyelitis virus causes leptomeningitis with a lymphocytic reaction. Histological examination of the spinal cord in this disease reveals perivascular lymphocytic cuffing in the acute stage, with death and phagocytosis of the infected motor neurones in the anterior horns. The axons of the dead motor neurones degenerate, which results in wasting of the anterior spinal roots and neurogenic atrophy of the muscles that they supplied (Hughes, 1966).

Syringomyelia

Syringomyelia classically presents with weakness and neurogenic atrophy of the small muscles of the hands. There is also loss of pain and temperature sensation in the hands. Clinically, the early lesion is localized mainly to the first thoracic segment of the cord.

The spinal cord is swollen and enlarged by an elongated central cavity (syrinx) which is most prominent in the lower cervical and upper thoracic regions but may extend into the brain stem; often the syrinx dissects posterolaterally into one dorsal horn of grey matter. In long-standing syringomyelia the central cavity is lined by a thick layer of gliosis. Damage to the pain and temperature fibres occurs as they cross the cord in close proximity to the syrinx. As the syringomyelic cavity enlarges, there is destruction of motor neurones in the anterior horns, with consequent axonal degeneration of motor fibres and neurogenic atrophy of the muscles that they supplied.

There is now a well-documented association between syringomyelia and bony abnormalities at the base of the skull. More recently, however, the correlation of syringomyelia with abnormalities involving the brain and spinal cord at the foramen magnum has become established (Appleby et al., 1968; Barnett, Foster and Hudgson, 1973). Some abnormalities include elongation and ectopia of the cerebellar tonsils (Chiari malformation) and adhesive thickening of the arachnoid around the foramen magnum and cisterna magna. Both lesions impair the flow of CSF from the fourth ventricle into the cisterna magna. It is thought that CSF is thus forced from the fourth ventricle into the central canal of the spinal cord. This probably causes hydromyelia at first, but the cavity enlarges, the ependymal lining of the canal splits and the syrinx assumes its familiar shape by the dissection of fluid into the cord (Williams and Weller, 1973). A more complete block in the CSF flow from the fourth ventricle may result in hydrocephalus.

Vascular disorders

Ischaemia and infarction of the spinal cord may occur if the spinal arteries are occluded by emboli or deprived of their blood supply by a dissecting aneurysm. In such cases there is destruction of the long tracts of the cord and the anterior horn cells in the area of infarction (Hughes, 1966). Lesser degrees of ischaemia may lead to transient sensory and motor symptoms, especially in the lower regions of the cord and cauda equina.

Thrombophlebitis of the spinal veins also causes destruction of the spinal cord, with loss of anterior horn cells, axonal degeneration in peripheral nerves and muscle wasting.

Multiple sclerosis

Multiple sclerosis plaques may occur in the spinal cord with demyelination of the involved tracts and relative sparing of the axons. In acute transverse myelitis there may be extensive demyelination of the motor fibres before they leave the spinal cord; this may lead eventually to axonal degeneration and chromatolysis of anterior horn cells.

Motor neurone disease

This term is usually reserved for a group of diseases with a wide spectrum of progressive upper and lower motor neurone paralysis involving the limbs and, in some cases, the cranial nerves. Four main types are described (Hughes, 1966; Liversedge and Campbell, 1974), viz. progressive muscular atrophy, amyotrophic lateral sclerosis, progressive bulbar paralysis and familial amyotrophic lateral sclerosis (Hirano, Kurland and Sayre, 1967).

The spinal cord is usually reduced in size and the anterior spinal roots are atrophic, particularly in the cervical region. Microscopic examination reveals varying degrees of axonal degeneration in the anterior and lateral corticospinal tracts and to a lesser extent in the spinocerebellar tracts (*Figure 46*). There is

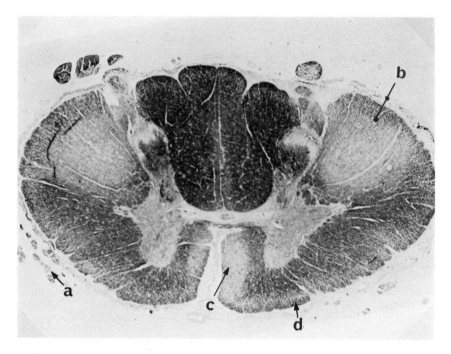

Fig. 46. T.S. thoracic spinal cord in amyotrophic lateral sclerosis showing atrophic anterior roots (a) and loss of myelin staining in the lateral (b) and anterior (c) cortico-spinal and spinocerebellar tracts (d). Luxol fast blue: Nissl stain. × 13

loss of anterior horn motor neurones, particularly in the posterolateral cell column; the cervical region is usually most severely affected. Degeneration of the axons from these cells is final: there is no regeneration, as the cell bodies are lost. There is wasting of the anterior spinal roots and neurogenic atrophy of muscles. Familial cases may show swelling and hyaline inclusions in the surviving anterior horn neurones. Sensory nerves, including the sural nerve, are usually unaffected in motor neurone disease, whereas loss of axons may be detected in the motor nerves. Muscle biopsies or autopsy specimens reveal neurogenic atrophy; surviving intramuscular nerves may show extensive collateral sprouting.

Spinal muscular atrophy

In this group of diseases there is degeneration of the motor neurones in the anterior horns of the spinal cord, and often non-specific chromatolytic changes in surviving neurones. Atrophy of the anterior spinal roots is seen and there is loss of large myelinated motor fibres from the mixed peripheral nerves. Neurogenic atrophy is the major change in affected muscles, but myopathic changes with death and regeneration of muscle fibres are also seen in the Kugelberg–Welander type of spinal muscular atrophy (Hausmanova-Petrusewicz, 1969; Dubowitz and Brooke, 1974).

There is considerable variation in the clinical presentation and prognosis in the spinal muscular atrophies which appear to have mainly an autosomal recessive pattern of inheritance (Emery, 1971). The patients present with muscle weakness: most commonly the proximal limb muscles are affected, but distal, bulbar, scapuloperoneal and faceoscapulohumeral involvement also occurs (Liversedge and Campbell, 1974). Sensory loss is seen only rarely.

Various types of spinal muscular atrophy can be distinguished by their age of onset and their speed of progression. The most acute form is Werdnig–Hoffman disease, first described in the 1890s. It has an estimated incidence of 1 in 20 000 births and a carrier frequency of from 1 in 60 to 1 in 80 in Britain (Pearn, Carter and Wilson, 1973); as such, it is one of the commonest recessive diseases of childhood. Severe generalized muscle weakness is usually seen by 3 months of age. The diaphragm and eye musculature may be spared. Tendon reflexes are absent and fasciculation in the affected muscles is indicative of anterior horn cell disease. The child usually dies within the first year, with severe loss of motor neurones and neurogenic muscular atrophy. A more slowly progressive form also occurs, with onset during the second year and death between 4 years and adolescence.

Kugelberg–Welander disease is a milder and more chronic form of spinal muscular atrophy, with mostly a recessive inheritance pattern. Signs of muscle weakness in the pelvic girdle usually appear from childhood to early adult life. Patients may still be able to walk 10 years after the onset of the disease and may live a normal life-span. In addition to the neurogenic atrophy in muscle biopsies, there are often myopathic features with death and regeneration of muscle fibres. Post-mortem studies reveal loss of anterior horn cells from the spinal cord (Gardner-Medwin, Hudgson and Walton, 1967).

Loss of anterior horn cells in the fetus is one of the causes of muscle weakness and deformities in arthro-gryposis multiplex congenita (Banker, Victor and Adams, 1957). In these cases the disease process may not progress after birth.

From the diagnostic standpoint it is important to distinguish the spinal muscular atrophies from muscular dystrophy. In the former, the muscle changes are mostly neurogenic atrophy, but the presence of myopathic changes in Kugelberg–Welander disease may lead to confusion with, for example, a very early case of Duchenne muscular dystrophy (Dubowitz and Brooke, 1973).

HEREDITARY PERIPHERAL NEUROPATHIES

A number of peripheral neuropathies have a definite hereditary basis. In some types of hereditary neuropathy, symptoms first become apparent in childhood or early adult life; in others the onset of symptoms occurs later. Mostly, the course of the neuropathy is slowly progressive and in many cases the patient's life-span is not significantly reduced despite severe disablement. Other systems and organs may be involved if the disease is a generalized metabolic abnormality. Where the disorder is confined to the nervous system, the brain and spinal cord may show pathological changes which may overshadow the peripheral nerve disorder. The diagnosis of a hereditary neuropathy is usually derived from the clinical features and family history of the disease, electrophysiological and biochemical investigations, and from the nerve or muscle biopsy findings.

There are a large number of hereditary neuropathies but they are uncommon and some are found only in small groups of families (Pratt, 1967). The neuropathies described in this section are those that occur most frequently, or those that have recognized metabolic basis. Inevitably, many of these neuropathies have eponymous names which often confuse any attempt at classification, but some effort has been made to explain the grouping used here.

Peroneal muscular atrophy and hypertrophic neuropathy

In this group of diseases there is slowly progressive neurogenic atrophy of muscles, particularly in the distal regions of the legs but also, in some cases, in the hands and distal parts of the arms. Where the disease is more generalized, the muscles of the back may be involved, which results in contracture and kyphoscoliosis. Sensory signs are present in some diseases in this group but they are usually less prominent than the motor defects. The pathology of the disorder varies. In some there is definite evidence of anterior horn cell loss with or without axonal degeneration in the corticospinal tracts of the spinal cord; in others there is hypertrophic change in the nerves with extensive segmental demyelination. Charcot, and Marie and Tooth in 1886 first described families with progressive distal muscle wasting and weakness involving the peroneal muscles and only later affecting the hands; their names are those commonly applied to this group of predominantly motor disorders. The classification followed here, however, is the result of clinical, electrophysiological and pathological studies by Dyck and Lambert (1968a,b) and includes the familial hypertrophic neuropathy described by Dejerine and Sottas (1893).

Charcot–Marie–Tooth disease with hypertrophic neuropathy and dominant inheritance

This is the commonest type of peroneal muscular atrophy and usually has an autosomal dominant pattern of inheritance, although sporadic cases do occur. The onset of symptoms is in the first and second decades. Pes cavus, foot weakness and disorders of gait occur early in the course of the disease, followed by progressive weakness and mild atrophy of the distal leg muscles,

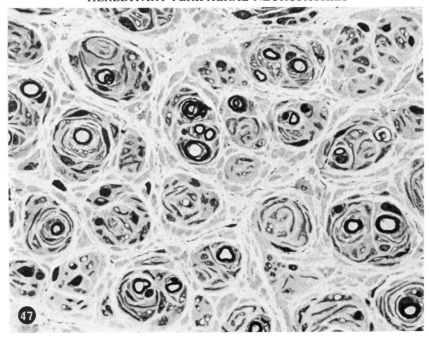

Fig. 47. Charcot–Marie–Tooth disease with hypertrophic neuropathy. T.S. sural nerve showing 'onion-bulb' whorls. 1 μm Araldite section stained with carbol fuchsin and toluidine blue. × 700

especially the peroneal group. Mild sensory impairment occurs late in the disease; it affects the distal parts of the limb and is less severe than the motor deficit. The hands are only slightly affected by the motor and sensory impairment.

A variable amount of clinical nerve hypertrophy is detectable and there is gross reduction in both sensory and motor nerve conduction velocities, with values of 5–20 m s^{-1} suggesting extensive segmental demyelination. CSF protein levels are usually normal. The disease has a progressive course but the outlook is usually favourable and confinement of the patient to a wheelchair is uncommon.

Pathology. The peripheral nerves are thickened, especially in the limbs, but, in the later stages, the spinal roots may also be hypertrophic (Symonds and Blackwood, 1962) and cause spinal cord compression. Histology reveals an increase in the transverse area of the nerve fascicles, onion-bulb whorls of hypertrophic neuropathy, segmental demyelination and loss of axons.

Biopsies of sural nerve and other sensory nerves in the lower limbs are useful for diagnostic purposes as they show the pathological features of the disease. The changes seen, however, do depend largely upon the severity and duration of the disease. Transverse sections of nerve show a variable and often severe loss of the large and small myelinated fibres. Onion-bulb whorls up to 20–30 μm in diameter are distributed throughout the nerve fascicles; some surround large myelinated fibres (*Figure 47*) and others have central demyelinated or thinly myelinated axons. Whorls devoid of myelinated fibres are also seen. Occasionally, clusters of small myelinated fibres are present in the whorls; they are similar to the clusters observed during axon regeneration (Ochoa and Mair, 1969). Non-myelinated fibres are probably reduced in number but they are mainly in groups separate from the onion-bulb whorls. Electron microscopy has shown that the majority of the cellular processes within the onion-bulb whorls are derived from Schwann cells; some contain individual non-myelinated axons and, occasionally, small myelinated axons. Although the endoneurial space is enlarged, the lakes of mucosubstance seen in some other types of hypertrophic neuropathy (Chapter 4) are not usually seen.

Teased-fibre studies (Dyck et al., 1970) reveal evidence of extensive segmental demyelination, but remyelination seems to occur promptly, so that only about 10 per cent of the internodes are devoid of myelin at any one time.

The presence of onion-bulb whorls strongly suggests that segmental demyelination is a major pathological process in the nerves in this disease. However, there is also progressive loss of large sensory and motor myelinated fibres. Dyck, Lais and Offord (1974) have shown that, in mild cases, the distal parts of the saphenous nerve have a greater loss of large myelinated fibres, a greater incidence of segmental demyelination and more onion-bulb whorls than the more proximal parts of the same nerve. They suggest that there is a primary defect in the neurones, with disordered axoplasmic transport and progressive atrophy of the distal ends of the nerves; the recurrent segmental demyelination and onion-bulb whorl formation may be secondary to axonal atrophy.

Muscle biopsies from the peroneal group or other affected muscles show neurogenic atrophy.

Dejerine–Sottas disease with hypertrophic neuropathy and recessive inheritance

Dejerine and Sottas (1893) described a brother and sister with a sensorimotor polyneuropathy and thickened nerves. The muscle wasting was more widespread than the distal peroneal group of Charcot–Marie–Tooth. Several families have now been described (Dyck and Lambert, 1968a; O'Brien, 1968), and the neuropathy probably has a recessive inheritance pattern. The onset of clinical signs begins in infancy or childhood, with delayed motor development and a slow progression of gait disturbance with ataxia. Muscle wasting, weakness and contractures are seen in the limbs; the patient may develop a kyphoscoliosis (O'Brien, 1968) and is usually unable to walk by the third decade of life. A progressive symmetrical glove and stocking sensory loss is also present. Marked enlargement of peripheral nerves is seen clinically, and the nerve conduction velocities are extremely low, suggesting extensive segmental demyelination. There is usually an increase in CSF protein levels.

Pathology. Motor and sensory nerves have an enlarged cross-sectional area; there is loss of large and small myelinated fibres, extensive segmental demyelination and remyelination together with the onion-bulb whorl formation of hypertrophic neuropathy (Dyck, 1966; Weller, 1967; Dyck and Gomez, 1968).

Transverse sections of sural nerve biopsies emphasize the increase in fascicular area and the severe loss of large and small myelinated fibres. Large-

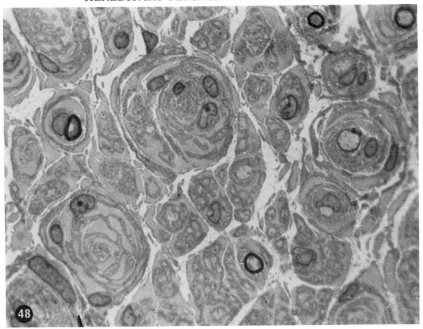

Fig. 48. T.S. sural nerve Dejerine–Sottas disease. The 'onion-bulb' whorls in this nerve are more complex than in Figure 47. Demyelinated and myelinated axons are seen. 1 μm Araldite section stained with carbol fuchsin and toluidine blue. × 1200

diameter (5–6 μm) demyelinated axons, devoid of myelin sheaths, are commonly seen and so are large remyelinating axons with thin myelin sheaths. The onion-bulb whorls are often larger than those in Charcot–Marie–Tooth hypertrophic neuropathy; they are more complex and are composed of multiple layers of imbricated cellular processes (Figure 48). Many whorls contain either demyelinated or remyelinating axons, whereas others have no axon at all at the centre. A number of fibres with thick myelin sheaths may be preserved and are usually separate from the onion-bulb whorls. Clusters of small regenerating nerve sprouts are not usually seen. The non-myelinated fibres are distributed throughout the nerve, either in small groups or within Schwann cells forming the whorls. An increase in mucoid material may be seen in the endoneurium; the vessels appear normal. In some cases the perineurium may be thickened.

Electron microscopy has shown that the majority of the cell processes in the whorls are derived from Schwann cells. Invagination of collagen bundles by the Schwann cells is frequently seen.

The extensive segmental demyelination is best seen in teased preparations; in many fibres practically the whole length of the axon is devoid of myelin. In teased specimens where osmium has not been used, the Schwann cell nuclei in the onion-bulb sheath surrounding the nerve can be demonstrated by haematoxylin staining.

Although the pathogenesis of the neuropathy in Dejerine–Sottas disease is uncertain, recurrent segmental demyelination with consequent onion-bulb whorl formation seems to be the major pathological process. Preliminary studies by Dyck *et al.* (1970) suggest that there may be a defect in the metabolism of ceramide hexoside lipids which could account for the apparently ineffective remyelination. Whether the eventual loss of large axons is secondary to the extensive segmental demyelination or due to primary involvement of the neurones in the disease process is unclear.

Neuronal type of Charcot–Marie–Tooth disease with dominant inheritance

The distribution of muscle weakness and wasting is very similar to the Charcot–Marie–Tooth disease with hypertrophic neuropathy described above, but there is more leg involvement, and the hands are less affected (Dyck and Lambert, 1968b). The onset of symptoms is not until middle age and the sensory impairment is mild compared with the motor loss. No enlargement of peripheral nerves is seen and the nerve conduction velocities are only slightly reduced. Electromyography shows denervation of muscles, particularly in the lower leg.

Pathology. Biopsies of sensory nerves reveal a very slight loss of the larger myelinated fibres due to axonal degeneration. No segmental demyelination or onion-bulb whorls are seen. A greater degree of axonal degeneration is seen in the motor nerves in the legs, and denervation atrophy can be detected in biopsies of the affected muscles. The site of the lesion may be in the motor axons or the anterior horn cells; very little change is seen in the posterior root ganglia.

Charcot–Marie–Tooth disease with progressive spinal muscular atrophy

This disease occurs sporadically with no well-defined pattern of inheritance. The onset is usually in the second and third decades, with profound symmetrical muscle wasting and weakness up to the mid-thigh region, followed by similar wasting of the hands and forearm (Dyck and Lambert, 1968b). There is no sensory abnormality or clinical enlargement of the nerves. Conduction velocities are normal or only moderately reduced, which suggests that there is little, if any, segmental demyelination. As the sensory nerves are clinically and electrophysiologically normal, there would be little histological abnormality in sural nerve biopsies. Muscle biopsy would confirm the denervation atrophy.

Infantile hypertrophic neuropathy

Cases of hypertrophic neuropathy occurring in infancy or early childhood have been described. Some are sporadic (Weller, 1967; Lyon, 1969), whereas others are familial (Joosten *et al.*, 1974). The children are hypotonic at birth; their motor development is retarded but there is relatively little muscle wasting. Sensory and motor nerve conduction velocities are either very slow or even unrecordable. Histologically, there is extensive segmental demyelination, with onion-bulb whorl formation (*Figure 49*); many of the large axons at the centre

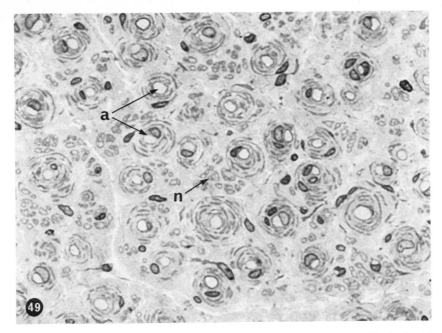

Fig. 49. *Infantile hypertrophic neuropathy. T.S. sural nerve showing 'onion-bulb' whorls with large axons (a) at their centres. Groups of truly non-myelinated axons (n) are also seen. 1 μm Araldite section stained with carbol fuchsin and toluidine blue. × 670*

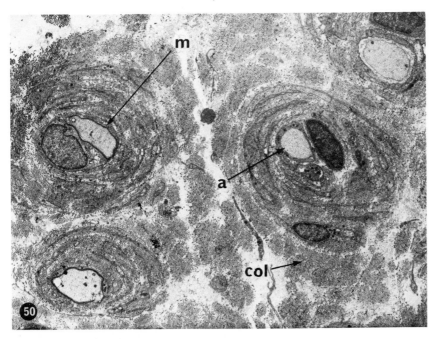

Fig. 50. *Infantile hypertrophic neuropathy. Electron micrograph of T.S. sural nerve showing thinly myelinated (m) or unmyelinated (a) large axons at the centre of 'onion-bulb' Schwann cell whorls. The collagen (col) in the nerve is increased. × 1800 (Courtesy J. Neurol. Neurosurg. Psychiat.)*

107

of the whorls have little or no myelin sheath (*Figure 50*). It is not at the moment clear how these cases fit nosologically into the hereditary hypertrophic neuropathies.

Friedreich's ataxia

Various hereditary ataxias have been described (Pratt, 1967), of which Friedreich's ataxia is the commonest. Cases are either sporadic or exhibit a recessive pattern of inheritance. Symptoms appear between the ages of 5 and 15 years with the onset of progressive ataxia, loss of reflexes and signs of corticospinal tract damage. The lower limbs are most severely affected; pes cavus and scoliosis are frequently seen. Nystagmus and dysarthria suggest a disturbance of cerebellar function affecting the cranial nerves. Muscle weakness and wasting may affect the hands, but sensory impairment is usually more widely spread and involves the distal parts of all four limbs. Patients may be confined to a wheelchair by the second or third decade. Nerve conduction studies reveal reduced action potentials in distal sensory nerves (Dyck and Lambert, 1968b) and significant slowing of motor nerve conduction (McLeod, 1971).

Pathology. The main pathological change in the peripheral nerves is the selective loss of large myelinated fibres from the sensory nerves due to axonal degeneration (Dyck et al., 1971). Atrophy of the dorsal spinal nerve roots is seen together with loss of sensory neurones from the posterior root ganglia (Hughes, Brownell and Hewer, 1968). Some segmental demyelination is seen but it is thought to be secondary to the primary axonal disease (Dyck and Lais, 1971). Small myelinated fibres in sensory nerves are preserved until late in the disease and the non-myelinated fibres appear to be unaffected.

At post-mortem the spinal cord is usually small and there is axonal degeneration, particularly in the fasciculus gracilis of the posterior columns. There is also some axonal loss from the corticospinal tracts and the posterior spinocerebellar tracts, although the cerebellum itself is usually normal. Degeneration of anterior horn cells is occasionally seen.

Patients with Friedreich's ataxia may die in heart failure due to fatty degeneration and fibrosis of the myocardium.

Hereditary sensory neuropathy

Ohta et al. (1973) have divided this group of disorders into four categories, which include:

Dominant hereditary sensory neuropathy

Many cases of sensory neuropathy with an autosomal dominant inheritance have been reported. The disease is a chronic progressive neuropathy with a dissociated sensory loss; the loss of pain and temperature sensation is out of proportion to the impairment of touch. Painless, relapsing ulcers appear on the toes and heels during the first two decades and may lead to the loss of digits (Schoene et al., 1970). The lower extremities are affected first and then the hands become involved; motor function is not altered until later in the disease. Death may occur as a result of uncontrolled infection or secondary amyloidosis.

Pathology. There is degeneration and loss of sensory neurones in the posterior root ganglia and degeneration of axons in the sensory nerves. The sacral roots and ganglia are affected first (Denny-Brown, 1951). Biopsies of sural nerve reveal a loss of small myelinated fibres initially; later the large myelinated fibres degenerate. The fibres that remain appear to be normal. Electron microscopy has shown that a large number of non-myelinated fibres are preserved; Schwann cell cords that presumably were once associated with myelinated fibres are also seen. Vacuolation of fibroblasts has been described as a prominent ultrastructural feature in this disease (Schoene *et al.*, 1970).

Recessive hereditary sensory neuropathy

In this disease the sensory deficit is already present at birth and is diffusely distributed over the body. Touch and pressure sensation are more severely affected than pain and temperature (Ohta *et al.*, 1973).

Pathology. There is a severe reduction in the number of myelinated fibres in sensory nerves to the skin; the non-myelinated fibres are depleted but to a lesser extent. Ballooned endoneurial fibroblasts have also been described in this disease (Ohta *et al.*, 1973).

Familial dysautonomia (Riley–Day syndrome)

A rare disorder which occurs in Jewish children and has an autosomal recessive inheritance. The disease is characterized clinically by widespread autonomic disorders which include defective lacrimation, postural hypotension, excessive sweating and gastro-intestinal hypermotility (Bannister, 1971). Most patients show dysphagia, aguesia, areflexia and a relative insensitivity to pain (Brain and Walton, 1969). The patients generally die in childhood from uraemia or chest infections.

Pathology. There appears to be an arrest of neuronal development in peripheral nerve ganglia due to a genetically determined functional defect in a nerve growth factor required for the normal growth and maturation particularly of sympathetic ganglia (see Chapter 3). Although the amount of nerve growth factor is raised in children with familial dysautonomia, it has a low functional binding activity (Siggers, 1975). Biopsies of sural nerves from these patients reveal a gross reduction in the non-myelinated axon population and no large myelinated fibres above 12 μm in diameter (Aguayo, Nair and Bray, 1971).

Peripheral neuropathies in disorders of lipid metabolism

The largest group of lipid disorders is the sphingolipidoses, in which there is accumulation of various types of sphingolipids, e.g. sphingomyelin, gangliosides, due to a deficiency of enzymes that metabolize these lipids. They are hereditary diseases often with a high incidence in Jewish populations. Most of the lipidoses affect the central nervous system much more severely than the peripheral nervous system, but patients with metachromatic leukodystrophy (sulphatide lipidosis) and Krabbe's globoid cell leukodystrophy have a significant defect of peripheral nerves. As the name 'leukodystrophy' implies, the structure and biochemistry of the myelin sheaths is disturbed in these diseases. Although Fabry's disease is also a disorder of sphingolipid metabolism, its main effect is upon blood vessels throughout the body.

The other disorders described in this section are associated with abnormalities of fatty acid metabolism (Refsum's disease) or lipoprotein synthesis.

Metachromatic leukodystrophy (sulphatide lipidosis)

This condition has an autosomal recessive inheritance pattern and derives its name from the accumulation of the lipid cerebroside sulphate in the brain, kidney and peripheral nerves. The lipid is metachromatic when stained by cresyl violet or thionine, i.e. it stains brown instead of the purple or blue colour of normal tissues.

The major effects of the disease are upon the central nervous system. Difficulty with walking may be noticed in the affected children at 2–3 years of age, with subsequent progressive paralysis and intellectual deterioration. Death usually occurs within 2 years of the onset of symptoms. There is a juvenile form with a later onset.

Peripheral nerve conduction velocities are greatly reduced in metachromatic leukodystrophy owing to the extensive segmental demyelination that occurs in both motor and sensory nerves.

Pathology. Sulphatide lipidosis is due to a deficiency of the enzyme arylsulphatase A (Austin *et al.*, 1966). This results in the accumulation of metachromatic lipid (cerebroside sulphate (sulphatide)) within neurones in the brain and peripheral ganglia but more especially in the white matter of the brain and within Schwann cells of peripheral nerves. Large amounts of the lipid are also found in renal tubular cells (*Figure 51*).

The accumulation of abnormal lipids is accompanied by extensive demyelination in the white matter and astrocytosis (Liu, 1968). Sural nerve biopsy in this disease shows loss of large-diameter myelinated fibres; there is very extensive segmental demyelination of the remaining nerves, with many thinly myelinated or demyelinated axons (*Figure 52*). Sulphatide deposits within the nerve can be stained metachromatically in frozen sections with cresyl violet or, more specifically, can be detected by Hollander's technique (Pearse, 1968), which stains the abnormal lipid orange. The sulphatide deposits within Schwann cells and endoneurial macrophages have a characteristic ultrastructure; each deposit is composed of groups of spherical or pyramidal inclusions about 1 μm in diameter (*Figures 52* and *53*). Some inclusions are lamellar, with a periodicity of 6 nm, but most characteristic are the stacks of discs with a 6 nm period (Gregoire, Perier and Dustin, 1966) formed from the polar sulphatide lipid separated by aqueous layers. (*Figure 54*). Some inclusions are seen in close association with myelin sheaths, which, although often thin, have a normal ultrastructure.

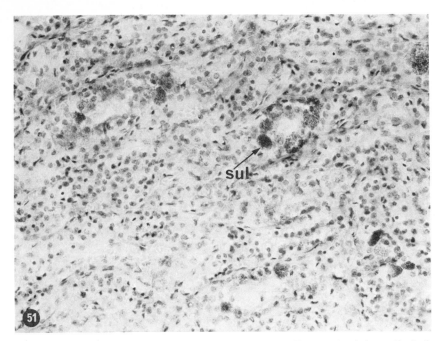

Fig. 51. Metachromatic leukodystrophy. Sulphatide in swollen renal tubular cells (sul). Hollander's stain; × 200

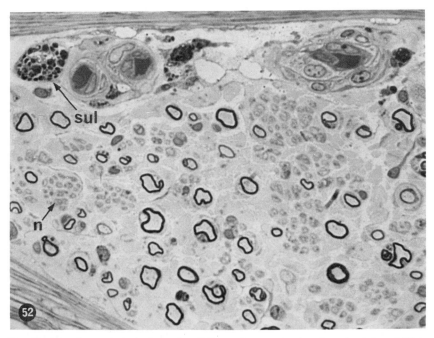

Fig. 52. Metachromatic leukodystrophy. T.S. sural nerve showing demyelinated and thinly myelinated (remyelinating) large axons. Non-myelinated axons (n). Sulphatide deposits (sul) are prominent in perivascular endoneurial macrophages (top left). 1 μm Araldite section stained with toluidine blue. × 790

111

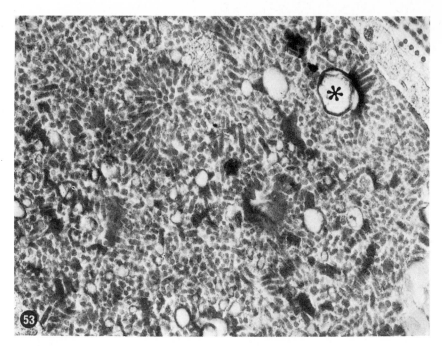

Fig. 53. Metachromatic leukodystrophy. Electron micrograph showing details of an intracellular sulphatide deposit. Much of the lipid is in rod- or disc-shaped bodies × 30 000. One area (*) is shown at higher magnification in Figure 54

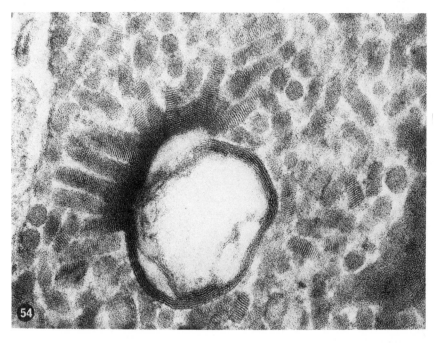

Fig. 54. Higher magnification of part of Figure 53 showing the sulphatide deposit as stacks of discs and in a lamellar form with a 5–6 nm periodicity. × 104 500

Diagnosis. Progressive dementia in a child with gross slowing of nerve conduction velocities would raise the suspicion of metachromatic leukodystrophy. Further diagnostic tests can be performed on the urine; either the centrifuged deposits can be examined for desquamated renal tubular cells containing metachromatic lipid (cresyl violet) or the urine can be tested for arylsulphatase A deficiency (Austin *et al.*, 1966). Decreased levels of arylsulphatase activity can be detected in fibroblasts in tissue culture (Kamensky *et al.*, 1973); this procedure together with the demonstration of metachromatic lipid in a peripheral nerve biopsy would confirm the diagnosis and it is rarely necessary to proceed to rectal biopsy or appendicectomy to examine autonomic ganglion cells, or to cerebral biopsy.

Krabbe's globoid cell leukodystrophy

Inherited as an autosomal recessive, the disease affects infants at 2–6 months of age. They fail to thrive, exhibit hypertonia and head retraction, and suffer from dysphagia, progressive mental deterioration and epilepsy. The children die in a decerebrate state by about 2 years of age. There is marked slowing of conduction, especially in the motor nerves in this disease, suggesting segmental demyelination (Dunn *et al.*, 1969).

Pathology. Extensive demyelination is seen in the white matter of the brain, together with an accumulation of mononuclear cells and large round multinucleate globoid cells from which the disease derives one of its names. There is an excessive amount of cerebroside lipid in the brain and the disease is probably due to a deficiency of cerebroside sulphotransferase which conjugates cerebroside with sulphate to form cerebroside sulphate (sulphatide) (Bachhawat, Austin and Armstrong, 1967).

Segmental demyelination is seen in the peripheral nerves, including the sural nerve (Dunn *et al.*, 1969). There is also an accumulation of crystalline deposits in Schwann cell cytoplasm with an increase in acid phosphatase activity. Foamy macrophages may be seen within the nerves but there is no large accumulation of lipid. Some degeneration of posterior root ganglion cells has been observed (Sourander and Olsson, 1968).

Fabry's disease (angiokeratoma corporis diffusum)

A sex-linked recessive hereditary disease where the affected hemizygous male develops skin lesions, dilated conjunctival vessels, corneal opacities, renal failure, cardiac complications and cerebral infarction. Although the patients often complain of spontaneous pains in the limbs related to changes in temperature, clinical evidence of peripheral neuropathy may not be found (Kocen and Thomas, 1970) and the nerve conduction velocities are normal.

Pathology. There is a deficiency of the enzyme ceramide trihexosidase in this disease and most of the renal, cardiac, cerebral and cutaneous manifestations are due either to deposition of the lipid, ceremide trihexoside in the tissue or to abnormalities of small arteries (Kahn, 1973). The histological diagnosis is usually made on skin biopsy. Sural nerve biopsies have shown a moderate reduction of myelinated fibres and the deposition of glycolipid (ceramide trihexoside) in the perineurium; the deposits have a lamellated ultrastructure with a 4 nm periodicity (Kocen and Thomas, 1970). Abnormal amounts of lipid are also found in the neurones of the myenteric plexus and in sympathetic ganglia.

Refsum's disease (heredopathia atactica polyneuritiformis)

First described by Refsum in 1946, this disease has an autosomal recessive pattern of inheritance with an onset of symptoms in early adult life. The condition is characterized by retinitis pigmentosa, cerebellar ataxia, ichthyosis, and nerve deafness (Steinberg et al., 1967). There is also a chronic progressive peripheral neuropathy with prominent distal muscle weakness and wasting, and symmetrical distal sensory loss. Peripheral nerves are slightly enlarged and nerve conduction velocities are reduced. The CSF protein levels are raised.

Raised levels of serum and tissue phytanic acid (a branched-chain fatty acid, 3,7,11,15-tetramethyl-hexadecanoic acid) were found in this condition by Klenk and Kahlke in 1963, and the disease is probably due to a failure of α-oxidation of phytanic acid (Steinberg et al., 1967). The abnormal fatty acid may form 50 per cent of total fatty acids in various organs, and improvement in symptoms has been obtained by dietary control of phytols (Steinberg et al., 1970).

Pathology. The peripheral nerves show the changes of hypertrophic neuropathy, with prominent onion-bulb whorl formation and segmental demyelination (Cammermeyer, 1956). There is often a severe loss of myelinated fibres, but in those that remain, myelination appears to be normal and the whorls contain one, two or three such fibres at the centre. Many non-myelinated fibres remain and some contain crystalline inclusions (Fardeau and Engel, 1969).

Disorders of lipoprotein

Tangier disease has an autosomal recessive inheritance pattern and is characterized by an absence of α-lipoprotein (high-density lipoprotein) in the blood and low serum cholesterol. The condition presents in childhood with characteristic large orange tonsils which contain excessive amounts of cholesterol ester. Similar lipid accumulation is seen in other organs. Some patients develop a progressive sensorimotor peripheral neuropathy with moderate slowing of nerve conduction velocities. Histologically, there is an accumulation of cholesterol esters within the Schwann cells and gross loss of myelinated and non-myelinated fibres due to axonal degeneration (Kocen et al., 1973). No segmental demyelination is seen.

A peripheral neuropathy also occurs in Bassen-Kornzweig's syndrome (Schwartz et al., 1963). This disease has an autosomal dominant inheritance and is characterized by serum β-lipoprotein deficiency. Various systemic and neurological disorders occur, including degeneration of the posterior columns, spinocerebellar tracts and anterior horn cells in the spinal cord (Mars et al., 1969).

Amyloidosis

Different types of amyloidosis can be distinguished, not only by their different clinical and pathological presentations, but also, to some extent, by the chemical nature of the amyloid deposit. In primary amyloidosis, where there is amyloid infiltration of tongue, heart, gut, smooth muscle, nerves and skin, and in amyloidosis associated with myeloma and other B-lymphocyte dyscrasias, the amyloid deposits are related to immunoglobulin light chains (Glenner *et al.*, 1971; Franklin, 1974). The amyloid that is found in liver, spleen, kidney and adrenals in secondary amyloidosis associated with chronic infections, rheumatoid arthritis, Hodgkin's disease, etc., is not related to immunoglobulin and is termed A-protein (Franklin, 1974). Similarly, the amyloid in familial amyloidosis is not related to immunoglobulin (Benson *et al.*, 1975).

Peripheral neuropathy is the main presenting feature in several autosomal dominant heredofamilial amyloid syndromes (Andrade *et al.*, 1970) and these will be described below. Neuropathy may also develop in patients with non-familial systemic amyloidosis as a result of amyloid infiltration of the nerve and its blood vessels or through compression of the median nerve due to amyloid infiltration of the flexor retinaculum (a carpal tunnel syndrome). These complications are mainly confined to patients with primary amyloidosis or with amyloidosis associated with malignant B-lymphocyte dyscrasias. Benson *et al.* (1975) found that 10 out of 87 patients with non-hereditary amyloidosis had evidence of peripheral neuropathy. Six had median nerve compression due to amyloid infiltration of the flexor retinaculum and four had either a diffuse sensorimotor or a pure sensory neuropathy. In the sensorimotor neuropathy amyloid deposits are seen in the endoneurium and in blood vessel walls (*Figure 55*); this distribution is similar to the Portuguese type of hereditary amyloidosis. Nerve fibre damage varies; in some cases there is extensive segmental demyelination (Benson *et al.*, 1975), whereas in others axonal degeneration is a prominent feature with selective loss of non-myelinated fibres. All the patients in Benson's series with a neuropathy had either a serum-M component or Bence-Jones protein. Neuropathy in patients with no evidence of monoclonal gammopathy is evidently much less common.

Although peripheral nerve involvement in secondary amyloidosis is much less frequent (Davies-Jones and Esiri, 1971; Dayan, Urich and Gardiner-Thorpe, 1971), amyloid may be seen in the walls of neural blood vessels.

Familial amyloidosis

There are three main types of autosomal dominantly inherited forms of amyloidosis where peripheral neuropathy is a prominent feature of the disease.

Portuguese familial amyloidosis (Andrade type)

First well documented in Portugal by Andrade in 1952, a similar disease has now been reported in other parts of the world especially in Japan (Andrade *et al.*, 1970). The onset of clinical symptoms is between 25 and 35 years of age and death from cachexia, infections, or renal failure occurs 7–10 years later.

There is early impairment of pain and temperature sensation, and autonomic disturbances, with anhidrosis, diarrhoea, sphincter disturbances, hypotension and impotence. Conduction studies (Dyck and Lambert, 1969) of nerves, *in vitro*, show a moderate reduction in the compound action potentials from A-delta (small myelinated) fibres and a virtual absence of C-fibre (non-myelinated) potential. This is consistent with the impairment of pain, temperature and autonomic function.

Pathology. Amyloid deposits are found in the kidneys and peripheral nerves and in other organs to a lesser extent. Biopsies of sensory peripheral nerves show large blobs of amyloid in the endoneurium and around blood vessels both in the endoneurium (*Figure 55*) and in the epineurium. The blobs stain with Congo red, which also makes them birefringent in polarized light. Electron microscopy reveals the typical non-branching 7–10 nm amyloid fibrils (Coimbra and Andrade, 1971). There is a very severe reduction or absence of non-myelinated fibres, and many empty Schwann cells are seen (Dyck and Lambert, 1969). The loss of small myelinated fibres is variable, but the large myelinated fibres may be well preserved.

The mechanism of this selective damage to non-myelinated and small myelinated fibres is difficult to determine. Neither compression of the nerve fibres by endoneurial amyloid deposits nor the effect of ischaemia through amyloid in blood vessel walls accounts for the selective degeneration of these fibres. Dyck and Lambert (1969) propose that the nerve fibre degeneration is a result of primary damage to the neurones in the posterior roots and autonomic ganglia, possibly due to amyloid deposition at these sites.

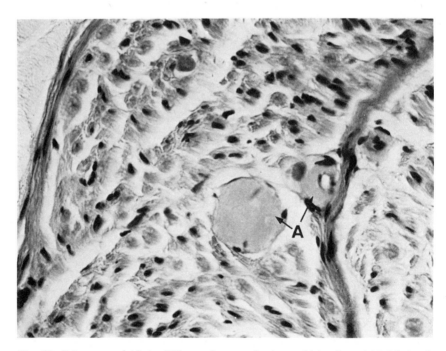

Fig. 55. Primary amyloidosis. T.S. sural nerve showing a blob of amyloid (A) in the endoneurium and amyloid in the wall of a small blood vessel. H. and E. stain; × 500

Indiana–Maryland familial amyloidosis (Rukavina type)

This disease has been described in a large kinship of Swiss and German origin in the USA (Andrade *et al.*, 1970). It is much less severe than the Portuguese type, and presents at about the age of 45 years with bilateral carpal tunnel syndrome and median nerve compression. Males are more severely affected than females. Later a progressive symmetrical polyneuropathy develops, affecting the legs more than the arms, with a loss of large myelinated fibres. There is little decrease in nerve conduction velocities.

Pathology. Widespread amyloid infiltration of blood vessel walls in many organs is seen; amyloid in the eyes causes vitreous opacities (Andrade *et al.*, 1970). Biopsies taken during the division of the flexor retinaculum for relief of nerve compression show amyloid infiltration of the retinaculum and the perineurial structures. The diagnosis of this disease may be made from histological examination of the retinaculum or gingival biopsies.

Iowa familial amyloidosis (van Allen type)

The main effects of this type of amyloidosis are upon the kidneys and peripheral nerves. A painful distal symmetrical sensorimotor polyneuropathy begins in the fourth decade and the patient usually dies within 20 years from renal disease. The neuropathy mainly affects the lower limbs, where there is muscle weakness and wasting, shooting pains and sensory impairment with early loss of pain sensation.

Pathology. Amyloid is seen mainly in the walls of the arterioles in the kidney. There is destruction of neurones in dorsal root ganglia and amyloid within the vessel walls of the posterior roots. Irregular masses of amyloid are also seen within the meninges (Adrade *et al.*, 1970).

Acute intermittent porphyria

In acute intermittent porphyria there is probably a defect in hepatic porphyrin metabolism. The disease has an autosomal dominant inheritance pattern with incomplete penetrance (Pratt, 1967). Attacks may be spontaneous or may be induced by drugs such as barbiturates, and take the form of severe episodes of abdominal pain, psychiatric disorders and peripheral neuropathy. During and after an acute episode there is an increased urinary excretion of porphyrin precursors, δ-amino-laevulinic acid and porphobilinogen, which may give the urine a 'port wine' colour.

The neuropathy is mainly motor in type and is characterized by flaccid paralysis and wasting of the proximal limb muscles, especially in the lower limbs (Ridley, 1969). Some sensory impairment may occur. Death may ensue, in the acute stages, from respiratory and bulbar paralysis. When recovery occurs, it progresses relatively slowly and may be incomplete (Heirons, 1957).

Pathology. Axonal degeneration is the major pathological change in the peripheral nerves. The distal ends of the large motor fibres in the intramuscular nerves of the proximal muscles are predominantly affected (Cavanagh and

Mellick, 1965). These changes are most effectively seen in thick frozen longitudinal sections of muscle stained with Sudan black or with silver stains which reveal the fragmentation of the intramuscular axons. Some loss of anterior horn cells is also seen (Heirons, 1957). In sensory nerves it is mainly the central processes passing into the spinal cord that degenerate. The pathology in this disease is considered to be a 'dying back' process (see p. 63) in which the distal ends of large nerves degenerate, although in acute porphyria it is not the longest fibres supplying distal musculature that are affected, as is usually the case in other 'dying back' neuropathies.

TRAUMATIC NERVE LESIONS

Most large peripheral nerves are well protected by muscle bulk but they may be injured by penetrating wounds, by the jagged edges of fractured bones or by the accidental intraneural injection of drugs. A number of superficial nerves are susceptible to direct injury—in particular, the lateral popliteal nerve at the head of the fibula and the ulnar nerve at the medial epicondyl.

As axonal degeneration usually occurs following direct nerve injury, the clinical effects are muscle denervation, together with sensory impairment and trophic changes in the skin. The pattern of clinical deficit varies with the site of nerve injury (Brain and Walton, 1969); the speed and degree of recovery decline the further the injury is from the site of innervation. As axon sprouts reinnervate the denervated areas, growing at an estimated 1–2 mm per day (Young, 1942), the nerve trunk distal to the site of injury becomes sensitive to stimulation. Deep sensibility followed by pain sensitivity are the first sensations to return to a denervated region (Brain and Walton, 1969). Temperature appreciation, fine touch and motor activity may subsequently return. Reinnervation of blood vessels and sweat glands can be tested by warming the skin. During the recovery period the denervated insensitive region requires protection from trauma and extremes of temperature. Passive movements of joints and electrical stimulation of denervated muscles help to retain mobility and reduce muscle atrophy.

Pathology. The pathology of axonal degeneration and regeneration following an uncomplicated nerve crush has been described in Chapter 4. As the axons in the distal stump of the nerve degenerate, the sensory end-organs that they supplied disappear and the denervated muscles atrophy. If the regeneration paths are blocked by scar tissue, or continuity of the nerve is lost, a traumatic neuroma may form (see Chapter 6, p. 145).

The functional regeneration of peripheral nerves following injury depends not only upon the ability of the nerve sprouts to grow out from the proximal stump of the axon, but also upon the anatomical continuity of the pathway to the site of innervation. Several grades of injury, of increasing severity, have been defined which take into account the degree of ultimate functional regeneration to be expected (Sunderland, 1968).

(1) Transient blockage of nerve conduction (neuropraxia). This usually follows compression of the nerve, and the largest fibres are affected most severely. As recovery begins within 2–3 weeks, the neural dysfunction is probably due to local segmental demyelination rather than axonal degeneration.

(2) Mild damage to the nerve resulting in axonal degeneration (axonotmesis) but with preservation of Schwann cell basement membrane and connective tissue continuity across the injured zone. Axon regeneration occurs at 1–2 mm per day and is usually effective unless the lesion is very proximal.

(3) More severe damage to the nerve causes severance of the axons and disorganization of the endoneurial connective tissue and Schwann cell basement membranes. However, the perineurium and fascicular structure may be preserved. Regeneration occurs but is not as effective as in (2).

(4) Severance of axons and disruption of endoneurial and perineurial connective tissue but with maintenance of anatomical continuity of the nerve. Regeneration in these cases is poorly orientated and less effective than in (3).

(5) If there is complete anatomical severance of the nerve, functional recovery is very unlikely to occur unless anatomical continuity can be restored.

Brain and Walton (1969) emphasized that the nature of the nerve lesion should be ascertained as soon as possible after the injury, by surgical exploration if necessary. The continuity of completely severed nerves may be restored either by suturing or by grafting; but if this procedure is delayed too long, little recovery occurs. Problems arise with grafting, especially if a large nerve is severed. Allografts have been used in animals, and reasonable success has been reported in cases treated with immunosuppressants (Pollard, McLeod and Gye, 1973). Experimental nerve allografts which have been allowed to undergo axonal degeneration within the donor prior to grafting, and thus have lost all their myelin, seem to stimulate a negligible immune response in the recipient (Das Gupta, 1967).

ENTRAPMENT AND COMPRESSION NEUROPATHIES

Focal muscle wasting or weakness and abnormal sensations may indicate the entrapment of a nerve or nerve root. This may occur in several situations. Nerve roots may be compressed in the intervertebral foramina by osteophytes in an osteoarthritic vertebral column, by acute intervertebral disc protrusions or by intraspinal tumours. More distally, individual nerves may suffer compression in fibro-osseous canals, as they pass through aponeuroses, or where they are in close association with swollen inflamed joints in rheumatoid arthritis or gout (Foster, 1974). In the arm the median nerve may be compressed at the wrist (carpal tunnel syndrome); the ulnar nerve most commonly suffers entrapment at the elbow as it passes through a canal formed by the origin of flexor carpi ulnaris and the medial epicondyle of the humerus. Posterior interosseous nerve compression may occur at the level of the supinator muscle in the arm (Lallemand and Weller, 1973). The common peroneal (Lateral popliteal) nerve is liable to be damaged by external compression at the neck of the fibula or may be compressed by an enlarged inflamed knee joint in rheumatoid arthritis.

Slowing of nerve conduction suggesting segmental demyelination commonly occurs at the site of compression in the carpal tunnel syndrome or ulnar nerve entrapment, and relief of the compression results in rapid recovery. In severe lesions there may be axon destruction, and recovery is slower and less complete.

Pathology. The nerve may be swollen and oedematous at the site of compression, and this often aggravates the entrapment. In mild cases of nerve compression, the major lesion is segmental demyelination (Aguayo, Nair and Midgley, 1971b; Neary and Eames, 1975), but in long-standing severe compression, axonal degeneration occurs. Onion-bulb whorls similar to those in hypertrophic neuropathy are seen in nerves subjected to repeated compression (Dyck, 1969) and in chronic human entrapment neuropathies (Neary and Eames, 1975); This suggests that the segmental demyelination is recurrent. Below the site of compression the fibre diameters and the thickness of the myelin sheaths are comparable with those of the nerve above the lesion. If axonal degeneration has occurred, clusters of regenerating fibres are seen in the nerve distal to the compression site. The nerve damage is thought to be caused mainly by ischaemia. In acute lesions caused by compression of the nerve by a tourniquet the myelin sheath is distorted in the large fibres at the edge of the tourniquet. Intersusseption of the paranodal myelin is followed by paranodal demyelination and a block in nerve conduction (Ochoa *et al.*, 1971).

NEUROPATHIES DUE TO VASCULAR DISEASE

Damage to peripheral nerves from ischaemia may be due to disease of the large arteries, particularly in the limbs, or to disorders that affect the small anastomosing vessels actually within the nerves. Mild ischaemic damage to nerves often results in primary segmental demyelination. If the ischaemia is severe, more axonal degeneration occurs which may be patchy and asymmetrical, depending upon the distribution of the vascular disease. The large myelinated fibres are generally affected early in the disease, then, with increasing severity of the ischaemia, the small myelinated fibres and finally the non-myelinated axons may degenerate.

The major effect of severe atherosclerosis of the large limb arteries is usually muscle ischaemia with intermittent claudication, and gangrene of the distal parts of the limb. However, over half of the patients with symptomatic arterial disease complain of paraesthesiae (Eames and Lange, 1967) and have evidence of peripheral neuropathy on clinical examination. The clinical picture of mononeuritis multiplex with asymmetrical motor and sensory nerve lesion is seen in many of the collagen diseases. Some 20–30 per cent of patients with polyarteritis nodosa have peripheral nerve involvement (Bleehen, Lovelace and Cotton, 1963). Similar neuropathies occur, but less frequently, in systemic lupus erythematosis (Johnson and Richardson, 1968), giant cell arteritis (Warrell, Godfrey and Olsen, 1968), scleroderma (Kibler and Rose, 1960) and Wegener's granulomatosis (Dyck, Conn and Okazaki, 1972); in some cases of diabetes (Raff and Asbury, 1968); and in patients with rheumatoid arthritis (Chamberlain and Bruckner, 1970) (see below). Vasculitis due to deposition of immune complexes within the vessel walls may involve peripheral nerves (*Figures 56* and *57*; Cream *et al.*, 1974).

Pathology. Severe loss of myelinated fibres from axonal degeneration may occur in nerves of limbs with chronic ischaemia due to atherosclerosis of large

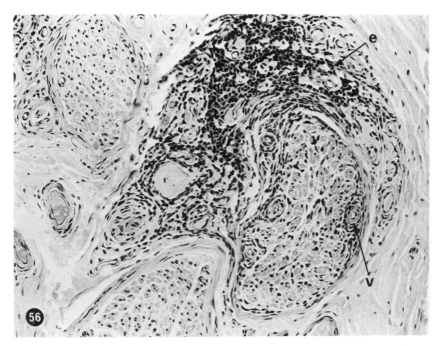

Fig. 56. Vasculitis and neuropathy in immune-complex cryoglobulinaemia. T.S. sural nerve showing lymphocyte infiltration of the epineurium (e) and around endoneurial blood vessels (v). H. and E. stain; × 200

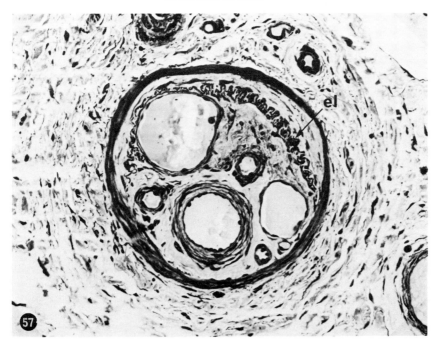

Fig. 57. Same nerve as Figure 56, showing revascularization of an epineurial artery. Old elastic lamina (el). Elastic stain; × 310

vessels (Garven, Gairus and Smith, 1962); some segmental demyelination may also be seen (Eames and Lange, 1967). In other diseases the nerve pathology is due mainly to vasculitis of the small vasa nervorum.

Owing to their patchy nature, vascular lesions may be missed in small biopsies of sural nerve. If the biopsies are to be examined, however, the whole thickness of the nerve should be taken, as the important epineurial blood vessels may not be included in fascicular biopsies. Dyck *et al.* (1972) examined vascular lesions in long lengths of limb nerve taken at post-mortem. They found that the pathology in the vessels was very similar in a range of diseases, including severe rheumatoid arthritis, polyarteritis nodosa, Churg–Strauss syndrome and Wegener's granulomatosis. Major lesions were found in the epineurial arteries, and consisted of perivascular mononuclear inflammatory cell infiltration and varying degrees of intimal proliferation and medial degeneration. Recent thrombi were seen in inflamed vessels. More chronic arterial lesions with proliferative endarteritis and revascularized arterial lumina were also seen in these diseases.

There is patchy and often total loss of nerve fibres in areas associated with vasculitis and vessel occlusion. Sometimes one fascicle may be affected more severely than another, or one part of a fascicle only may be devoid of nerve fibres. In acute lesions axon and myelin breakdown may be seen at the site of the vascular occlusion or vasculitis, and distal to it. Examination of distal parts of the nerve in chronic lesions may reveal no vessel pathology but only the cumulative effect of patchy axonal degeneration throughout the length of the nerve.

Rheumatoid neuropathy

Neuropathies that occur in a proportion of patients with rheumatoid arthritis have been devided into three main groups (Chamberlain and Bruckner, 1970).

(1) Compression or entrapment neuropathies associated with early rheumatoid arthritis and local joint changes. The median nerve at the wrist, the ulnar nerve at the elbow and the common peroneal nerve at the knee are most frequently involved.

(2) Distal sensory neuropathies occur in benign rheumatoid arthritis. There is a patchy glove and stocking sensory impairment and minimal motor weakness. Nerve conduction studies either are normal or show marked slowing indicative of segmental demyelination (Chamberlain and Bruckner, 1970). Sural nerve biopsies from patients in this group show either primary segmental demyelination or moderate axonal degeneration (Weller, Bruckner and Chamberlain, 1970).

(3) Severe fulminating sensorimotor neuropathies are found in patients with severe malignant rheumatoid arthritis. Rheumatoid factor is present in high titre and evidence of vasculitis is seen in the nail beds and elsewhere. There is a severe distal motor weakness, especially in the feet, and electromyography reveals extensive denervation (Chamberlain and Bruckner, 1970). Acute vasculitis is seen in the nerves from these severely affected patients (Dyck *et al.*, 1972); the inflammation is

associated with deposits of immune complexes (IgG, IgM and Complement) in the vessel walls (Conn, McDuffie and Dyck, 1972). More chronic vascular lesions show intimal thickening which contain no immune complexes. There is extensive loss of large and small myelinated fibres from the nerves due to axonal degeneration; many of the non-myelinated axons may also degenerate (Weller *et al.*, 1970).

NEUROPATHIES DUE TO TOXIC SUBSTANCES

A number of organic and inorganic substances have been shown to cause peripheral neuropathies in man and experimental animals. The neuropathy may be the major lesion or it may accompany damage to the central nervous system. Most toxic neuropathies occur either as a result of exposure to organic or inorganic substances used in industry or following the administration of a drug; certain bacterial toxins also cause peripheral neuropathies. A few of the substances that cause neuropathies are listed in *Table 3*; a more complete list has been compiled by the World Federation of Neurology (Walton, 1968).

TABLE 3
Some substances causing peripheral neuropathies

(1) *Organic substances*	(a) Industrial:	
		Triorthocresyl phosphate (TOCP)
		Acrylamide
		p-bromophenylacetylurea
		Carbon disulphide
		Diethylthiocarbamate, etc.
		Organic mercury compounds
	(b) Drugs:	
		Isoniazid
		Nitrofurantoin
		Sulphonamides
		Cloroquine
		Vinca, alkaloids, thalidomide, phenytoin, streptomycin, etc.
		Alcohol
(2) *Inorganic substances*		Arsenic
		Mercury
		Antimony
		Thallium
		*Lead
(3) *Bacterial toxins*		Botulinum
		Tetanus
		*Diphtheria

* Lead and diphtheria, in particular, cause segmental demyelinating neuropathies.

Most substances that have a selective action upon the nervous system affect the neurones more severely than the glia or Schwann cells. This is particularly so with the peripheral nervous system, where the distal ends of long, large-diameter axons degenerate, which produces a 'dying back' neuropathy (Cavanagh, 1973). Lead salts and diphtheria toxin are the only well-documented substances in cases where the major effect in peripheral nerves is upon Schwann cells and where primary segmental demyelination is the major pathological feature.

Axonal degeneration in toxic neuropathies

A typical 'toxic' peripheral neuropathy is seen in organophosphorus poisoning (Cavanagh, 1973). Alkyl phosphates are very toxic owing to their potent anticholinesterase action, but it is the less toxic aryl phosphates, e.g. triorthocresyl phosphate (TOCP), which cause peripheral neuropathies. TOCP itself is not toxic, but it is metabolized by the liver to form a toxic agent (Cavanagh, 1973). Although the major effects of TOCP poisoning are upon the motor system, the onset of symptoms is marked by abnormal sensations, such as tingling, particularly in the feet. Following this, motor weakness develops in the feet and later in the legs, giving rise to a high stepping gait and ataxia. The neurological signs progress for the first 2 weeks and then remain stationary.

Morphologically, the peripheral nerve damage is seen mainly in the intramuscular nerves. Fifty-μm sections of muscle stained with Sudan black for myelin or silver stains for axons reveal axonal degeneration of the distal ends of large-diameter fibres. Sensory nerves show widespread degeneration, especially in the distal limb regions; the annulospiral endings of the muscle spindles are most severely affected. Once a fibre has started to degenerate at the distal end, the axon continues to 'die back' for some distance. 'Dying back' neuropathies derive their name from this phenomenon of progressive degeneration from the distal end towards the cell body that occurs particularly in large-diameter nerve fibres. Axonal degeneration is rarely found in the main nerve trunks, most of the damage being confined to the intramuscular branches. Electron microscopy has revealed axonal changes above the site of degeneration; these consist mainly of an accumulation of angulated membrane profiles and some dense bodies (Prineas, 1969a). The pattern of degeneration suggests that the metabolism of the neurone is affected and that the cell can no longer support distal parts with long axonal processes. However, this hypothesis has been very difficult to substantiate experimentally (Bradley and Williams, 1973).

After about 2 weeks signs of regeneration appear. Collateral sprouting of surviving fibres and, later, regeneration of the damaged axons occurs. If administration of the toxic material ceases, regeneration of the nerves may be virtually complete, especially if the 'dying back' process has not progressed too far proximally. During the regeneration phases the neurone cell bodies of affected axons show the changes typical of the chromatolysis that usually accompanies axonal regeneration; no other more specific neuronal changes are seen.

The 'dying back' phenomenon is also seen in spinal cord tracts in TOCP poisoning. There is axonal degeneration at the rostral end of long ascending pathways in the cord and at the caudal ends of the corticospinal tracts (Cavanagh and Patangia, 1965). In this respect, the fibre damage resembles the changes found in Friedreich's ataxia, a hereditary 'dying back' condition (see p. 108). Regeneration of central pathways is not usually very effective.

Other industrial toxins cause 'dying-back' neuropathies but there is some variation in the pattern of pathological change. In some cases the central nervous system damage overshadows the peripheral neuropathy.

Acrylamide, which is used widely in the polymer industry, causes a 'dying back' neuropathy in man and animals (Fullerton and Barnes, 1966) with ataxia and distal limb weakness. Early pathological changes are seen in the Pacinian corpuscles in the feet. These are followed by degeneration of the annulospiral endings around muscle spindles and later by 'dying back' of motor nerve endings supplying extrafusal muscle fibres (Schaumburg, Wisniewski and Spencer, 1974). Degeneration of axon terminals is seen also in the gracile nuclei of the spinal cord (Prineas, 1969b). Regeneration of peripheral nerve terminals and recovery occurs if the exposure to acrylamide ceases.

Thallium, used in rat and ant killers, causes a polyneuritis of the 'dying back' type, with painful sensory symptoms (Cavanagh et al., 1974).

Certain therapeutic agents may produce a 'dying back' peripheral neuropathy, e.g. thalidomide (Fullerton and O'Sullivan, 1968), isoniazid (Ochoa, 1970) and Vinca alkaloids (Bradley et al., 1970). Isoniazid is detoxicated by acetylation in the liver; this process is fairly rapid in the majority of the population. Some patients, however, owing to a recessively inherited trait, inactivate isoniazid only slowly, so that high blood levels of the drug are reached. It is these patients who develop the, mainly motor, isoniazid neuropathy with damage to both myelinated and non-myelinated fibres (Ochoa, 1970). The main effect of isoniazid seems to be upon vitamin B_6 metabolism, and the administration of pyridoxal or pyridoxamine protects the patient from the toxic effect of the drug (Cavanagh, 1973). Vinca alkaloids, used in the treatment of leukaemia, may cause a neuromyopathy; one of the effects of these agents is interference with axoplasmic flow.

Alcoholics may develop a peripheral neuropathy which is essentially similar to the 'dying back' neuropathy of thiamine (vitamin B_1) deficiency (see p. 127).

Botulinum toxin (type A) causes paralysis due to a block in neuromuscular transmission. The nerve terminals do not degenerate, but, after a variable delay, they start to sprout and form nerve–muscle contacts (Duchen, 1971).

Segmental demyelination in toxic neuropathies

Some toxic substances affect mainly the Schwann cells in peripheral nerves and produce a primary segmental demyelinating neuropathy. The two main agents concerned are diphtheria toxin and lead. Diphtheria toxin is produced by *Corynebacterium diphtheriae* bacilli that are infected with a bacteriophage. The toxin may diffuse from the site of injection in the pharynx and cause a generalized sensorimotor neuropathy (Fisher and Adams, 1956), with slowing of conduction velocities. Recovery is rapid and usually complete. Binding of the toxin is very rapid, but there is a latent period before the onset of clinical signs and of segmental demyelination within the nerve. The small myelinated fibres are affected most severely, as paranodal myelin breakdown spreads to involve the whole internode. In larger fibres the myelin breakdown is often confined to the paranodal regions (Cavanagh and Jacobs, 1964) and is best seen in teased nerve preparations. The toxin appears to inhibit protein and lipid synthesis; thus, the early changes seen at the nodes of Ranvier suggest that these may be active sites of myelin production and repair, and therefore suffer early when there is a block in Schwann cell metabolism (Cavanagh, 1973).

Deaths from lead poisoning are now rare, and the peripheral neuropathy may be minor compared with the central nervous system signs. Much of the information about the pathology of lead neuropathy has therefore been obtained from experimental animals. Fullerton (1966) showed a reduced conduction velocity in the nerves of guinea-pigs chronically poisoned by lead salts. Segmental demyelination and severe axonal degeneration was found in most nerves throughout the body, and no particular fibre size was selectively affected. The electron microscopic features of lead neuropathy have been described by Lampert and Schochet (1968).

METABOLIC NEUROPATHIES

Some of the metabolic neuropathies, including amyloid neuropathy, have already been discussed in the section on hereditary neuropathies. Under the present heading the neuropathies associated with diabetes are numerically the most important, although in some areas of the world neuropathies due to vitamin deficiencies are also prominent. Uraemic neuropathies have become more important as patients with chronic renal failure survive longer with haemodialysis. Neuropathies also occur in some other endocrine disorders.

Diabetic neuropathy

The commonest type of neuropathy associated with diabetes mellitus is a distal, symmetrical, predominantly sensory polyneuropathy. Symptoms and sensory signs occur to a significant degree in about 5 per cent of patients (Bruyn and Garland, 1970), probably more often in poorly controlled diabetes of long duration. Patients complain of numbness and paraesthesiae of the toes and feet, and, later, of the fingers. There is often a burning sensation in these regions and pains in the calves. A reduction in nerve conduction velocity is frequently found in the limb nerves, and nerve biopsies reveal primary segmental demyelination (Thomas and Lascelles, 1966). Onion-bulb whorls, typical of hypertrophic neuropathy, have been described in diabetic neuropathy (Ballin and Thomas, 1968), which suggests that recurrent segmental demyelination occurs. Axonal degeneration is seen in more chronic diabetic neuropathies. The exact pathogenesis of the neuropathy is uncertain; it may be partly due to accompanying vascular disease, but, as occluded vessels are not invariably found (Thomas and Lascelles, 1966), a primary metabolic disorder affecting Schwann cell metabolism cannot be excluded.

A more acute proximal mononeuritis multiplex may occur in diabetes, but it is less common. Pathological studies in this disease have revealed multiple occlusions of the small blood vessels (vasa nervorum) in the nerve resulting in localized infarcts of nerve and axonal degeneration (Raff and Asbury, 1968).

There may be autonomic dysfunction in diabetes, with impotence in the male, diarrhoea, sphincter disturbances and postural hypotension. These disorders appear to be due to degeneration of autonomic ganglia (Hensley and Soergel, 1968).

126

Neuropathies due to vitamin deficiencies

Apart from vitamin B_{12} deficiency, neuropathies due to lack of vitamins usually occur in conditions of malnutrition or malabsorption. The deficiencies are usually multiple and may include several vitamins together with other nutrients. Beriberi, due to vitamin B_1 (thiamine) deficiency, and pernicious anaemia (B_{12} deficiency) are two disorders which show prominent changes in the peripheral nerves. A more comprehensive survey of deficiency neuropathies has been compiled by Erbslöh and Abel (1970).

The neuropathy of thiamine (B_1) deficiency is a 'dying back' neuropathy resembling that of triorthocresyl phosphate poisoning (Cavanagh, 1973). It is either a mixed sensorimotor, mainly sensory or mainly motor neuropathy, affecting the distal parts of the limbs, the feet more often than the hands. Axonal degeneration at the distal ends of the nerves predominates, and recovery is slow and incomplete if the vitamin deficiency is long-standing. Thiamine pyrophosphate is an important co-enzyme in carbohydrate metabolism, and lack of this vitamin causes an accumulation of pyruvate and lactate. The heart may be affected and cardiac failure may ensue.

Vitamin B_{12} deficiency is usually due to loss of intrinsic factor in the gastric mucosa resulting in poor absorption of vitamin B_{12} from the gut. Intestinal parasites, ileal resection and dietary deficiencies may also result in vitamin B_{12} deficiency. Clinically, the central nervous system signs of subacute combined degeneration of the spinal cord predominate, and the disease is usually associated with pernicious anaemia. There is progressive axonal degeneration in the corticospinal tracts and the dorsal columns of the spinal cord. Degeneration of the long tracts is most severe at their distal ends, i.e. rostral end of the ascending tracts and caudal end of the descending tracts. Many patients also have signs of a peripheral neuropathy with paraesthesiae in the hands and feet. Conduction velocities in the peripheral nerves are only marginally reduced. Clinical features and pathological studies suggest that it is a 'dying back' neuropathy affecting the large myelinated fibres most severely (McLeod, Walsh and Little, 1969).

Uraemic neuropathy

The introduction of dialysis treatment for chronic renal failure has resulted in the much longer survival of patients with deficient renal function. Many such patients develop a chronic distal symmetrical neuropathy which is predominantly sensory but may have a significant motor component. Seventy-five per cent of the patients with chronic renal failure examined by Thomas et al. (1971) had pain, numbness and paraesthesiae, mainly in the feet, which improved with adequate treatment by dialysis. The cause of the neuropathy is not clear. Pathological studies reveal predominantly axonal degeneration in the distal portions of sensory nerves (Dyck et al., 1971; Thomas et al., 1971), particularly involving the larger fibres. In sural nerve biopsies, taken from different levels in uraemic patients, Dyck et al. (1971) found only 4 per cent degenerating fibres at mid-calf level but 51 per cent degenerating fibres at the ankle. Furthermore, there was segmental demyelination in the more proximal biopsy. They concluded that the sensory neurone was primarily affected, which gave rise to degeneration of the distal end of the axon, and that the segmental demyelination proximally was secondary and due to alterations in the axon.

Neuropathies in endocrine disorders

Hyperthyroidism affects mainly muscle, producing a periodic paralysis syndrome. Myxoedema with hypothyroidism, however, may produce either an entrapment neuropathy involving the median nerve at the wrist or a diffuse polyneuropathy (Dyck and Lambert, 1970). This latter neuropathy is associated with a reduction in the conduction velocity of large and small myelinated fibres, with primary segmental demyelination. Improvement of the clinical symptoms and increase in conduction velocities occurs as thyroid hormone is replaced.

Peripheral neuropathies occur in acromegaly, although they are mostly due to entrapment. Segmental demyelination, in addition to axonal degeneration, has been reported in a more widespread neuropathy associated with this disease (Dinn, 1970).

Amyloidosis (see p. 115)

INFLAMMATORY DISORDERS OF PERIPHERAL NERVES

Pathological changes are seen in peripheral nerves in a variety of inflammatory disorders. Local involvement of nerves by the spread of pyogenic infections and abscess formation often results in axonal degeneration and subsequent scarring and fibrosis of the nerve. More generalized inflammatory disorders, however, present as polyneuropathies or involve several individual nerves.

Acute post-infectious polyneuritis (Guillain–Barré syndrome) is seen following a variety of acute viral infections and after surgical operations. It is basically an allergic segmental demyelinating neuropathy with the features of a delayed hypersensitivity reaction very similar to experimental allergic neuritis. The neuropathies that are encountered in measles, rubella, smallpox, mumps, chickenpox and infectious mononucleosis, and after smallpox and rabies vaccination, are probably of this type (Brain and Walton, 1969). In other infections the viruses attack the neurones directly, and involve either the dorsal root ganglion cells (e.g. herpes zoster) or the anterior horn cells and lower motor neurones of the brain stem (e.g. poliomyelitis; see p. 98).

Peripheral nerves are specifically involved in leprosy. The causative agent, *Mycobacterium leprae*, spreads along the peripheral nerves as well as through the blood stream in lepromatous leprosy; a more localized, granulomatous lesion is seen in the nerves in tuberculoid leprosy.

Granulomata may cause thickening of peripheral nerves in sarcoidosis, a disease which can affect any part of the nervous system or muscles (Matthews, 1965). Other organs are usually more severely affected, but a muscle biopsy is often useful in establishing the diagnosis.

Peripheral neuropathies are not usually a feature of protozoal infections, but a polyneuropathy or mononeuritis may be seen in chronic malaria.

Inflammatory disorders involving the vessels in peripheral nerves are discussed in the section on vascular disease.

Guillain—Barré syndrome (acute post-infective polyneuritis)

Acute post-infective polyneuritis is the commonest form of acute neuropathy in Britain. It is seen predominantly in males between the ages of 20 and 50 years, but it can occur at any age in either sex (Brain and Walton, 1969). There is often a history of a virus infection 2—4 weeks before the onset of symptoms, although other precipitating events, such as surgical procedures, have been recorded (Arnason and Asbury, 1968). The course of the disease is variable: it may be an acute, chronic or relapsing illness (Widerholt, Molder and Lambert, 1964; Thomas et al., 1969; Prineas, 1972). There is often sensory loss and paraesthesiae in the feet and hands in the early stages of the disease, but motor signs usually predominate. Widespread paralysis may occur very rapidly, affecting the proximal and distal limb muscles. Weakness of the pharyngeal and respiratory muscles often makes tracheostomy and artificial ventilation necessary. The paralysis may last for 1—4 weeks or longer and then gradual recovery occurs over the next 3—6 months; 3—6 per cent of patients relapse. Recovery from the motor paralysis is usually good if the patient survives the acute stages, but a proportion of cases are left with residual muscle weakness, especially if they were severely paralysed during the attack (Bradley, 1974). Typically, the CSF protein level is raised but the cell content is low. Peripheral nerve conduction velocities in the limbs are often reduced by 50 per cent during the paralytic phase, but they may be normal if only the nerve roots are involved in the disease process.

Pathology. Post-mortem studies of patients dying in the acute stages of the disease reveal congestion of the meninges and petechial haemorrhages in the spinal cord. Chromatolysis of anterior horn cells and dorsal root ganglia may be seen together with some round cell infiltration around blood vessels. The main pathological changes, however, are seen in the nerve roots and peripheral nerves, especially those containing motor fibres.

The primary pathological lesion of Guillain—Barré polyneuropathy is allergic segmental demyelination; it is very similar to experimental allergic neuritis (see Chapter 4). If the demyelination is mild, neural function returns with remyelination and, as the axons are preserved, recovery may be complete. In severe cases of the disease there is often extensive axonal degeneration within the affected nerves. This may result in chromatolysis of motor and sensory neurones, denervation atrophy of muscle and a poor functional recovery.

Examination of paraffin sections reveals widespread infiltration of the affected nerve fascicles by macrophages, lymphocytes and plasma cells.

The inflammatory cells are seen both around endoneurial blood vessels and between the individual nerve fibres. Myelin breakdown associated with the inflammatory exudate is best-demonstrated in longitudinal sections. Isolation of individual fibres in teased preparations reveals segmental demyelination and remyelination with varying amounts of axonal degeneration, depending upon the severity of the disease. Electron microscope studies of post-mortem (Wisniewski *et al.*, 1969) and biopsy material (Prineas, 1972) from patients with Guillain–Barré syndrome have revealed the cellular mechanisms involved in the demyelination. Macrophages, which constitute 80 per cent of the inflammatory cell infiltrate in the nerve, penetrate the basement membranes surrounding the nerve fibre and extend cytoplasmic tongues to displace the Schwann cell cytoplasm away from the myelin sheath. Stripping of the myelin sheath from around the axon and the breakdown of the myelin debris is mediated chiefly by macrophages in the presence of small lymphocytes. The Schwann cell seems to play little part in the destruction of the sheath (cf. primary demyelination in diphtheritic neuropathy—Chapter 4). Demyelinated axons may be observed in the acute stages of the neuropathy; they are devoid of a myelin sheath, but often they are surrounded by a thin layer of Schwann cell. Remyelination occurs in a similar manner to that seen in other demyelinating neuropathies (see Chapter 4). Axons are, at first, encompassed by a thin myelin sheath which is gradually increased in thickness. Short lengths of axon may be remyelinated by the longitudinal extension of the adjacent myelin sheath (Prineas, 1972).

In the ultrastructural studies quoted there was little axonal degeneration. However, in other accounts of the histology in the Guillain–Barré syndrome axonal degeneration has been observed in peripheral nerves, and neurogenic atrophy has been described in the muscles (Arnason and Asbury, 1968).

Hypertrophic changes have been described in the nerves of patients with recurrent Guillain–Barré polyneuritis (Prineas, 1972; Dolman and Allen, 1973). Inflammatory cells are associated with the onion-bulb whorls that surround demyelinated and remyelinating axons; these appearances resemble chronic, relapsing, allergic neuritis (Thomas *et al.*, 1969).

Although the exact aetiology of Guillain–Barré polyneuritis is not known, it has the features of a cell-mediated delayed hypersensitivity reaction. It is very similar to experimental allergic neuritis, in which sensitivity to peripheral nerve myelin is induced by the injection of peripheral nerve protein. The mechanism of sensitization in Guillain–Barré syndrome is unclear, but it is possibly a reaction to a preceding viral infection.

Virus infections

Poliomyelitis (see p. 98) and herpes zoster are the major viral diseases which directly involve the peripheral nervous system.

Herpes zoster (varicella zoster)

Herpes zoster is due to an acute infection involving primarily the first sensory neurone and the area of skin that it supplies. The infecting agent is the virus *Varicella zoster*, which is closely related to chickenpox virus and is distinct from herpes simplex virus.

Usually, herpes zoster occurs in patients over 50 years of age; it often complicates a debilitating illness but does also present in otherwise healthy individuals (Brain and Walton, 1969). It may be due to recrudescence of a latent infection with chickenpox virus; when due to reinfection, it has an incubation period of about 2 weeks. The disease presents as a papular and vesicular rash in the skin supplied by the nerves from one or several sensory ganglia; there are often prodromal symptoms of burning or shooting pains and hyperalgesia in the area of skin involved. As thoracic dorsal root ganglia are typically affected, the skin rash often follows a narrow, band-like distribution around one side of the chest wall, thus marking the affected dermatome. Involvement of the sensory ganglia of cranial nerves occurs, especially the trigeminal, and again the rash delineates the skin supplied by the nerve. Only rarely is the disease bilateral; occasionally, *Varicella zoster* causes an encephalitis, myelitis, or polyneuropathy (Dayan, Ogul and Graveson, 1972). The rash fades after a few days, with scarring and frequently some loss of sensation in the affected area. Persistent pain (post-herpetic neuralgia) may be a problem.

Pathology. In the acute stages of herpes zoster the affected sensory ganglia are swollen, congested and haemorrhagic. Infarction due to thrombotic occlusion of blood vessels within the ganglia may also occur. The upper cervical and thoracic posterior root ganglia are most frequently affected, but usually only on one side. Necrotic and shrunken ganglion cells are seen; some are vacuolated and there may be neuronophagia. There is perivascular infiltration of mononuclear cells and occasionally polymorphonuclear cells are present. The inflammation may extend into the spinal cord or posterior root and, to a minor extent, into the anterior root (Hughes, 1966). Fibrosis of the ganglion and axonal degeneration follow the death of the sensory neurones.

Varicella zoster does not remain viable for very long in post-mortem tissue and has not been isolated from sensory ganglia and grown in tissue culture. However, the virus has been identified by electron microscopy and by direct immunofluorescence within the affected neurones of the trigeminal ganglion in acute herpes zoster. *Varicella zoster* has also been detected in the cytoplasm and nuclei of the perineurial cells and Schwann cells of the trigeminal nerve, but not within the axons (Esiri and Tomlinson, 1972). The skin lesions of herpes zoster show acantholysis and vesicles in the epidermis. Epidermal cells contain nuclear inclusions (*Figure 58*) which are visible with the light microscope and contain *Varicella zoster* virus. Electron microscopy reveals virus both in the nucleus and in the cytoplasm (*Figure 59*). The virus nucleoid, in the nucleus of the cell, may be seen as a dense dot or as an open circle surrounded by one outer layer, with a total diameter of 70—80 nm (*Figure 59*). In the cytoplasm, or outside the cell, the complete virus has an additional membrane coat derived from the host's cell membrane and has a total diameter of about 140 nm. Individual virus particles may be isolated from the skin vesicle fluid and viewed in the electron microscope as negatively stained preparations. Virus in the neurones and Schwann cells has a similar morphology to virus particles in the skin.

One of the unanswered questions in herpes zoster is whether the virus remains latent in the skin or in the ganglion cell. Esiri and Tomlinson (1972) concluded from their studies that the virus might spread along the nerve in the endoneurial cells, especially the Schwann cells but not in the axons. Other viruses are also transported from the periphery to the neurone cell body (Kristensson and Olsson, 1973) but except in rabies, varicella zoster, and perhaps herpes simplex, the neural spread of viruses seems to be an unimportant route of dissemination in man (Johnson and Mims, 1968).

131

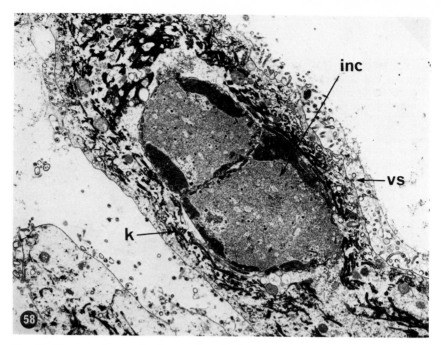

Fig. 58. Electron micrograph of an epidermal cell in herpes zoster, showing pale nuclear inclusions (inc). Densely staining keratin (k) is seen in the cytoplasm. There are many virus particles (vs) in the extracellular spaces. ×6750

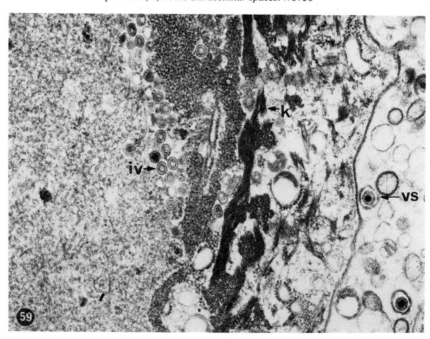

Fig. 59. Higher magnification of part of Figure 58 showing incomplete varicella zoster virus in the nucleus (iv) and the complete virus in the extracellular space (vs). Cytoplasmic keratin (k). ×40 000

132

Leprosy

Leprosy is a very widespread disease in subtropical and tropical zones, affecting 15 million people or more, throughout the world (Manson-Bahr, 1966); it is particularly common in Africa. The disease is caused by an acid-fast bacillus, *Mycobacterium leprae*, which probably spreads by contagion in overcrowded conditions; children are more susceptible to leprosy than adults. *Mycobacterium leprae* is $0.2-0.5$ μm in diameter and $1.5-5$ μm in length. It has not been cultured *in vitro* but can be transmitted to experimental animals (Rees and Waters, 1971).

The type of leprosy which develops depends upon the immunological responsiveness of the patient. There are two major stable forms, i.e. lepromatous and tuberculoid leprosy, with at least three categories of intermediate or borderline type (Ridley, 1973); peripheral nerves are affected in all types.

The *lepromatous* type is characterized by macular lesions on the skin which are not hypoaesthetic (Lever, 1967). Bacilli spread quickly from the skin to other parts of the body in the blood, and many patients with lepromatous leprosy have an almost constant bacteraemia. Dissemination of leprous bacilli also occurs as they pass along peripheral nerves. The characteristically widespread distribution of the infection in lepromatous leprosy is thought to reflect the lack of resistance or hypersensitivity to *M. leprae*. Intradermal injection of an extract of killed leprous bacteria (lepromin test) causes little reaction in these patients, whereas a granuloma forms in patients with tuberculoid leprosy.

Tuberculoid leprosy is characterized by well-defined anaesthetic depigmented macules on the skin. As the larger peripheral nerves become involved in the disease, there is increasing loss of sensation; trophic ulcers develop in anaesthetic areas, and digits may be lost. The nerves become nodular and thickened, but other organs are not affected. The hypersensitivity and resistance to *M. leprae* in the tuberculoid form is reflected in the positive lepromin test, in which a granuloma is produced following intradermal injection of an extract of killed leprosy bacteria.

Borderline leprosy and intermediate types of the disease have features of both main types.

Pathology. In *lepromatous leprosy* there is destruction of skin appendages and infiltration of the dermis by macrophages, lymphocytes and plasma cells; large foamy 'lepra' cells containing the weakly acid-fast *M. leprae* are also seen (Ridley, 1973). Nerves in the skin may exhibit only minor changes. Larger peripheral nerves are usually heavily invaded by leprous bacilli but show little inflammation, and the general architecture of the nerve is maintained. Extensive axonal degeneration occurs, and, in advanced cases, the nerves are replaced by hyalinized connective tissue. Miliary granulomas are seen in many organs, including lymph nodes, spleen, bone marrow and testis. Light and electron microscope studies of epoxy resin-embedded nerve biopsies from patients with lepromatous leprosy have shown a gross reduction in the number of non-myelinated axons in the early stages of the disease (Yoshizumi and Asbury, 1974) and a loss of large myelinated fibres (Dastur, Ramamohan and Shah, 1973). Groups of leprous bacilli are seen within Schwann cells, particularly those associated with non-myelinated fibres; the Schwann cells

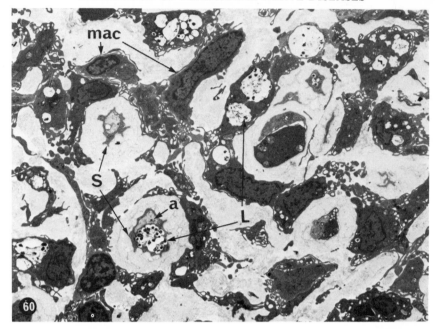

Fig. 60. Borderline leprosy. A low-power electron micrograph showing epithelioid macrophages (mac) in the endoneurium. They surround Schwann cells (S) which contain non-myelinated axons (a). Leprous bacilli (L) in macrophages and Schwann cells. × 2800 (Courtesy of Dr R. King)

appear to actively phagocytose the organisms (Dastur *et al.*, 1973). Bacilli are also seen within the axons; again, the non-myelinated fibres are most frequently involved (Yoshizumi and Asbury, 1974). The organism may spread along the axon or there may be transference of the bacilli from one Schwann cell to another. As one injected Schwann cell dies and bursts, other Schwann cells may phagocytose the organisms. Axonal degeneration is a prominent feature of this disease and is probably a result of infection of Schwann cells and axons by the mycobacteria.

Figures 60 and *61* show the electron microscope appearances in a case of borderline leprosy. There was severe loss of large, myelinated fibres from many of the fascicles in this nerve and a reduction in non-myelinated fibres. Large numbers of macrophages are seen in the nerve (*Figure 60*), often elongated and epithelioid in form. Mycobateria are found within Schwann cells, many of which still surround non-myelinated axons (*Figure 61*). The bacteria are also observed within macrophages.

Tuberculoid leprosy is characterized by granulomatous lesions which resemble sarcoid (Lever, 1967). Histiocytes become epithelioid in character, and, together with giant cells and lymphocytes, form granulomata in the dermis of the skin and erode epidermis (Ridley, 1973). Cutaneous nerves are destroyed, which produces anaesthetic lesions in the skin. A few *M. leprae* are present in tuberculoid lesions. The peripheral nerves are nodular and thickened owing to the tuberculoid granulomata which destroy the normal architecture of the nerve. Segmental demyelination and axonal degeneration is seen in the

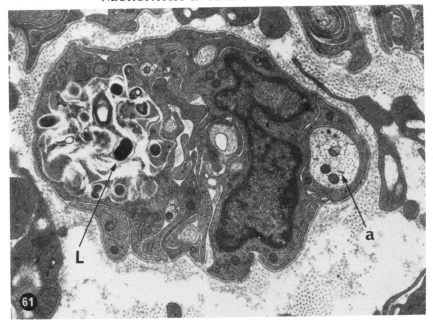

Fig. 61. Same case as Figure 60, showing a Schwann cell containing leprous bacilli (L). Axon (a). × 13 040 (Courtesy of Dr R. King)

involved nerves (Job, 1973), but few lepra bacilli are present in the Schwann cells. Gradually the nerves are destroyed and replaced by granulomatous tissue and severe fibrosis, which makes regeneration impossible (Finlayson, Bilbao and Lough, 1974). Other organs are not usually involved in tuberculoid leprosy.

NEUROPATHY IN MALIGNANT DISEASE

The central and peripheral nervous systems are commonly damaged by primary and metastatic tumours, but it is now well recognized that neurological lesions may also occur as a remove effect of malignant disease (Brain and Norris, 1965). Myopathies are probably the commonest non-metastatic effects of tumours, and they often present before the neoplasm itself is obvious. Myasthenic syndromes, encephalopathies, myelopathies, and peripheral neuropathies also occur; they may similarly precede the appearance of the tumour.

Metastatic involvement of the nervous system often complicates carcinoma of the lung and breast, etc. Secondary deposits in the spine frequently result in compression of the spinal cord or nerve roots, with varying degrees of axonal loss from peripheral nerves. Local infiltration of nerves by tumour may occur, as, for example, when an apical carcinoma of the lung invades the brachial plexus. Leukaemic or carcinomatous deposits in the meninges may cause cranial nerve lesions due to local infiltration. The tumour cells invade the

135

perineurium and the endoneurium, causing axonal degeneration and segmental demyelination (Kashef and Das Gupta, 1967; Henson and Urich, 1970).

Non-metastatic effects of cancer on the nervous system include a variety of encephalopathies. Some are due to virus infections, e.g. progressive multifocal leukoencephalopathy, whereas others are a result of nutritional deficiencies, e.g. Wernicke's encephalopathy in patients with gastric carcinoma.

Encephalomyelitis has been described in association with oat-cell carcinoma of the lung, with widespread inflammatory lesions in the hippocampus, the brain stem, spinal cord and posterior root ganglia (Henson and Urich, 1970). Death of neurones and lymphocytic infiltration is seen histologically; as a result of the destruction of motor and sensory neurones, axonal degeneration occurs within the peripheral nerves. The neurological symptoms may precede the discovery of the tumour by up to 3 years.

Peripheral neuropathies associated with malignant disease are seen mostly in patients with bronchial carcinoma, but also with carcinomas of stomach, breast, pancreas and colon (Henson and Urich, 1970). The neuropathy is often combined with a myopathy or cerebellar disorder (Croft, Urich and Wilkinson, 1967). Three main types of neuropathy have been distinguished by Croft *et al.* (1967): (1) a mild peripheral neuropathy which is often a terminal feature of malignant disease; (2) a severe, subacute or acute crippling sensorimotor polyneuropathy, which may precede the discovery of the tumour; (3) a relapsing neuropathy similar to (2). Histological studies of involved nerves have shown a variable loss of axons in the severe sensorimotor neuropathy and in some cases a significant degree of segmental demyelination (Croft *et al.*, 1967). Focal lymphocytic infiltration of the nerves is seen, which suggests that the nerve fibre damage may be due to an immunological mechanism.

PERIPHERAL NEUROPATHIES IN THE AGED

Peripheral nerve disorders of varying severity are seen in older people. This is partly due to neuropathies accompanying vascular disease and malignant tumours, both of which occur more frequently in older age groups. Recurrent trauma to peripheral nerves throughout life may also play a part in the impairment of peripheral nerve function. Histological studies have shown fine structural changes in Schwann cells with ageing (Weller, 1967; Ochoa and Mair, 1969). Teased-fibre preparations may reveal evidence of previous segmental demyelination and axonal degeneration in older patients, particularly in exposed nerves such as the sural nerve (Lascelles and Thomas, 1966; Arnold and Harriman, 1970). Care must be taken, therefore, in establishing histological controls in various age groups so that 'wear and tear' damage in peripheral nerves of older patients is not mistaken for evidence of a specific neuropathy.

AUTONOMIC NEUROPATHIES

The autonomic nervous system is affected in a number of peripheral neuropathies (Johnson and Spalding, 1974). Autonomic involvement in diabetes, Fabry's disease, familial amyloid and dysautonomia have already been discussed in this chapter, and the pathology in these diseases has also been reviewed by Thomas (1973). Neurological disorders of the gastro-intestinal tract cover a wide field, and the pathology of the myenteric plexus has been reviewed by Smith (1970).

Other lesions of the autonomic nervous system are rare and only sometimes limit the life-span of the patient (Bannister, 1971). Cases of acute pan-dysautonomia have been described with postural hypotension and loss of thermo-regulator reflexes and sudomotor activity (Thomashefsky, Horwitz and Feingold, 1972). Small regenerating non-myelinated axons have been described in the sural nerve following recovery from an autonomic neuropathy (Appenzeller and Kornfeld, 1973). The cause is unknown. The Shy–Drager syndrome is a more severe condition, with postural hypotension, defective sweating and sphincter disturbances linked with signs of basal ganglia disease and Parkinsonian features. Both the parasympathetic and sympathetic systems are affected, and patients may die from cerebral ischaemia during a hypotensive episode (Bannister, 1971). There are different varieties of the disease but all point to a multiple-system atrophy. Pathologically, there is neuronal atrophy, particularly of the autonomic efferent neurones in the in-termediolateral columns of the spinal cord (Graham and Oppenheimer, 1969).

MYASTHENIA GRAVIS

Myasthenia gravis is a specific muscle disease characterized by an abnormal amount of weakness of voluntary muscle following repetitive contraction or prolonged tension; the muscles recover their power after a period of inactivity. The most frequent age of onset of the disease is about 20 years, and females are affected more than males. The symptoms are attributed to a defect in neuromuscular transmission.

Pathology. Isolated muscle fibre damage with foci of lymphocytic infiltration may be seen in patients with myasthenia gravis (Russell, 1953) and there may be some neurogenic atrophy (Brownell, Oppenheimer and Spalding, 1972). Intravital methylene blue staining has shown disordered and bizarre terminal arborizations of the intramuscular nerves, and ultrastructural studies reveal simplification of the cleft pattern of the motor end-plates (Woolf, 1966; Engel and Santa, 1971).

In addition to the changes in the muscles, many patients with myasthenia gravis have abnormalities in the thymus ranging from the anomalous occurrence of germinal centres in the thymic cortex to thymomas (Simpson, 1974).

Recent immunological studies (see Gutmann and Chou, 1976) have produced clear evidence in myasthenia gravis of cellular and humoral immunological reactions to acetylcholine-receptor protein. This could reduce the number and possibly the sensitivity of acetylcholine receptors at the motor end-plates and result in the clinical physiological and pharmacological features of the disease.

REFERENCES

Aguayo, A. J., Nair, C. P. V. and Bray, G. M. (1971a). 'Peripheral nerve abnormalities in the Riley–Day syndrome.' *Arch. Neurol. (Chicago)*, **24**, 106.

Aguayo, A., Nair, C. P. V. and Midgley, R. (1971b). 'Experimental progressive compression neuropathy in the rabbit.' *Arch. Neurol. (Chicago)*, **24**, 358.

Andrade, C., Araki, S., Block, W., Cohen, A. S., Jackson, C. E., Kuroiwa, Y., McKusick, V. A., Nissim, J., Sohar, E. and Van Allen, M. W. (1970). 'Hereditary amyloidosis.' *Arthritis Rheumat.*, **13**, 902.

Appenzeller, O. and Kornfeld, M. (1973). 'Acute pandysantonomia: clinical and morphological study.' *Arch. Neurol. (Chicago)*, **29**, 334.

Appleby, A., Foster, J. B., Hankinson, J. and Hudgson, P. (1968). 'The diagnosis and management of the Chiari abnormality in adult life.' *Brain*, **91**, 131.

Arnason, B. G. and Asbury, A. K. (1968). 'Idiopathic polyneuritis after surgery.' *Arch. Neurol. (Chicago)*, **18**, 500.

Arnold, N. and Harriman, D. G. F. (1970). 'The incidence of abnormality in control human peripheral nerves studied by single axon dissection.' *J. Neurol. Neurosurg. Psychiat.*, **33**, 55.

Austin, J., Armstrong, D., Shearer, L. and McAfee, D. (1966). 'Metachromatic form of diffuse cerebral sclerosis. VI. A rapid test for sulphatase A deficiency in the urine.' *Arch. Neurol. (Chicago)*, **14**, 259.

Bachhawat, B. K., Austin, J. and Armstrong, D. (1967). 'A cerebroside sulphotransferase deficiency in a human disorder of myelin.' *Biochem. J.*, **104**, 15c.

Ballin, R. H. M. and Thomas, P. K. (1968). 'Hypertrophic changes in diabetic neuropathy.' *Acta. Neuropath. (Berlin)*, **11**, 93.

Banker, B. Q., Victor, M. and Adams, R. D. (1957). 'Arthrogryposis multiplex due to congenital muscular dystrophy.' *Brain*, **80**, 319.

Bannister, R. (1971). 'Degeneration in the autonomic nervous system.' *Lancet*, **ii**, 175.

Barnett, H. J. M., Foster, J. B. and Hudgson, P. (1973). *Syringomyelia*. London; Saunders.

Benson, M. D., Cohen, A. S., Brandt, K. D. and Cathcart, E. S. (1975). 'Neuropathy, M components, and amyloid.' *Lancet*, **i**, 10.

Bleeren, S. S., Lovelace, R. E. and Cotton, R. E. (1963). 'Mononeuritis multiplex in polyarteritis nodosa.' *Quart. J. Med.*, **32**, 193.

Bradley, W. G. (1974). 'The neuropathies.' In *Disorders of Voluntary Muscle*. Ed. by J. N. Walton. Edinburgh; Churchill Livingstone.

Bradley, W. G. (1975). In *Disorders of Peripheral Nerves*. Oxford; Blackwell.

Bradley, W. G., Lassman, L. P., Pearce, G. W. and Walton, J. N. (1970). 'The neuromyopathy of vincristine in man: clinical electrophysiological and pathological studies.' *J. Neurol. Sci.*, **10**, 107.

Bradley, W. G. and Williams, M. H. (1973). 'Axoplasmic flow in axonal neuropathies. I. Axoplasmic flow in cats with toxic neuropathies.' *Brain*, **96**, 235.

Brain, W. R. and Norris, F. (1965). In *The Remote Effects of Cancer on the Nervous System*. New York; Grune and Stratton.

Brain, W. R. and Walton, J. N. (1969). In *Brain's Diseases of the Nervous System*, 7th edn. London; Oxford University Press.

Brewis, M., Poskanzer, D. C., Rolland, C. and Miller, H. (1966). 'Neurological disease in an English city.' *Acta Neurol. Scand. Suppl.*, **24**, 1.

Brownell, B., Oppenheimer, D. R. and Spalding, J. M. K. (1972). 'Neurogenic muscle atrophy in myasthenia gravis.' *J. Neurol. Neurosurg. Psychiat.*, **35**, 311.

Bruyn, G. W. and Garland, H. (1970). 'Neuropathies of endocrine origin.' In *Handbook of Clinical Neurology*, Vol. 8, p. 29. Ed. by P. Vinken and G. W. Bruyn. Amsterdam; North-Holland.

Buchthal, F. and Rosenfalck, P. (1973). 'On the structure of motor units.' In *New Developments in Electromyography and Clinical Neurophysiology*, Vol. I, pp. 71–85. Ed. by J. E. Desmedt. Basle; Karger.

Calne, D. B. and Pallis, C. A. (1972). 'Electromyography and nerve conduction studies.' *Br. J. Hosp. Med.*, June, 775.

Cammermeyer, J. (1956). 'Neuropathological changes in hereditary neuropathies. Manifestations of the syndrome heredopathia atactica polyneuritiformis in the presence of interstitial hypertrophic polyneuropathy.' *J. Neuropath. Exp. Neurol.*, **15**, 340.

Cavanagh, J. B. (1973). 'Peripheral neuropathy caused by chemical agents.' *C.R.C. Critical Reviews in Toxicology*, November, 365.

138

REFERENCES

Cavanagh, J. B., Fuller, N. H., Johnson, H. M. and Rudge, P. (1974). 'The effects of thallium salts with particular reference to the nervous system changes. A report of three cases.' *Quart. J. Med.*, **43**, 293.

Cavanagh, J. B. and Jacobs, J. M. (1964). 'Some quantitative aspects of diphtheritic neuropathy.' *Br. J. Exp. Pathol.*, **45**, 309.

Cavanagh, J. B. and Mellick, R. S. (1965). 'On the nature of the peripheral nerve lesions associated with acute intermittent porphyria.' *J. Neurol. Neurosurg. Psychiat.*, **28**, 320.

Cavanagh, J. B. and Patangia, G. N. (1965). 'Changes in the central nervous system in the cat as a result of tri-*o*-cresyl phosphate poisoning.' *Brain*, **88**, 165.

Chamberlain, M. A. and Bruckner, F. E. (1970). 'Rheumatoid neuropathy.' *Ann. Rheumat. Diseases*, **29**, 609.

Coimbra, A. and Andrade, C. (1971). 'Familial amyloid polyneuropathy: an electron microscope study of the peripheral nerve in five cases. I. Interstitial changes.' *Brain*, **94**, 199.

Conn, D. L., McDuffie, F. C. and Dyck, P. J. (1972). 'Immunopathologic study of sural nerves in rheumatoid arthritis.' *Arthritis Rheumat.*, **15**, 135.

Cream, J. J., Hern, J. E. C., Hughes, R. A. C. and MacKenzie, I. C. K. (1974). 'Mixed or immune complex cryoglobulinaemia and neuropathy.' *J. Neurol. Neurosurg. Psychiat.*, **37**, 82.

Croft, P. B., Urich, H. and Wilkinson, M. (1967). 'Peripheral neuropathy of sensorimotor type associated with malignant disease.' *Brain*, **90**, 31.

Das Gupta, T. K. (1967). 'Mechanisms of rejection of peripheral nerve allografts.' *Surg. Gynecol. Obstet.*, **125**, 1058.

Dastur, D. K., Ramamohan, Y. and Shah, J. S. (1973). 'Ultrastructure of lepromatous nerves. Neural pathogenesis in leprosy.' *Int. J. Leprosy*, **41**, 47.

Davies-Jones, G. A. and Esiri, M. M. (1971). 'Neuropathy due to amyloid in myelomatosis.' *Br. Med. J.*, **2**, 444.

Dayan, A. D., Ogul, E. and Graveson, G. S. (1972). 'Polyneuritis and herpes zoster.' *J. Neurol. Neurosurg. Psychiat.*, **35**, 170.

Dayan, A. D., Urich, H. and Gardiner-Thorpe, C. (1971). 'Peripheral neuropathy and myeloma.' *J. Neurol. Sci.*, **14**, 21.

Dejerine, J. and Sottas, J. (1893). 'Sur la névrite interstitielle, hypertrophique et progressive de l'enfance.' *Compt. Rend. Soc. Biol.*, **45**, 62.

Denny-Brown, D. (1951). 'Hereditary sensory radicular neuropathy.' *J. Neurol. Neurosurg. Psychiat.*, **14**, 237.

Dinn, J. J. (1970). 'Schwann cell dysfunction in acromegaly.' *J. Clin. Endocrinol. Metab.*, **31**, 140.

Dolman, C. L. and Allen, B. M. (1973). 'Relapsing hypertrophic neuritis.' *Arch. Neurol. (Chicago)*, **28**, 351.

Dubowitz, V. and Brooke, M. H. (1973). In *Muscle Biopsy: A Modern Approach*. London; Saunders.

Duchen, L. W. (1971). 'An electron microscope study of the changes induced by Botulinum toxin in the motor end-plates of slow and fast muscle fibres of the mouse.' *J. Neurol. Sci.*, **14**, 47.

Dunn, H. G., Lake, B. D., Dolman, C. L. and Wilson, J. (1969). 'The neuropathy of Krabbe's infantile cerebral sclerosis (globoid cell leukodystrophy).' *Brain*, **92**, 329.

Dyck, P. J. (1966). 'Histological measurements and fine structure of biopsied sural nerve: normal, and in peroneal muscular atrophy, hypertrophic neuropathy and congenital sensory neuropathy.' *Mayo Clin. Proc.*, **41**, 742.

Dyck, P. J. (1969). 'Experimental hypertrophic neuropathy. Pathogenesis of onion-bulb formations produced by repeated tourniquet applications.' *Arch. Neurol. (Chicago)*, **21**, 73.

Dyck, P. J., Conn, D. L. and Okazaki, H. (1972). 'Necrotizing angiopathic neuropathy. Three-dimensional morphology of fiber degeneration related to sites of occluded vessels.' *Mayo Clin. Proc.*, **47**, 461.

Dyck, P. J., Ellefson, R. D., Lais, A. C., Smith, R. C., Taylor, W. F. and Van Dyke, R. A. (1970). 'Histologic and lipid studies of sural nerves in inherited hypertrophic neuropathy: preliminary report of a lipid abnormality in nerve and liver in Dejerine–Sottas disease.' *Mayo Clin. Proc.*, **45**, 286.

Dyck, P. J. and Gomez, M. R. (1968). 'Segmental demyelinization in Dejerine–Sottas disease.' *Mayo Clin. Proc.*, **43**, 280.

Dyck, P. J., Johnson, W. J., Lambert, E. H. and O'Brien, P. C. (1971a). 'Segmental demyelination secondary to axonal degeneration in uraemic neuropathy.' *Mayo Clin. Proc.*, **46**, 400.

REFERENCES

Dyck, P. J. and Lais, A. C. (1971). 'Evidence for segmental demyelination secondary to axonal degeneration in Friedreich's ataxia.' In *Clinical Studies in Myology*, Part 2, p. 253. International Congress Series 295. Amsterdam; Excerpta Medica.

Dyck, P. J., Lais, A. C. and Offord, K. P. (1974). 'The nature of myelinated nerve fibre degeneration in dominantly inherited hypertrophic neuropathy.' *Mayo Clin. Proc.*, **49**, 34.

Dyck, P. J. and Lambert, E. H. (1968a). 'Lower motor and primary sensory neuron diseases with peroneal muscular atrophy. I. Neurologic, genetic and electrophysiologic findings in hereditary polyneuropathies.' *Arch. Neurol. (Chicago)*, **18**, 603.

Dyck, P. J. and Lambert, E. H. (1968b). 'Lower motor and primary sensory neuron diseases with peroneal muscular atrophy. II. Neurologic, genetic and electrophysiologic findings in various neuronal degenerations.' *Arch. Neurol. (Chicago)*, **18**, 619.

Dyck, P. J. and Lambert, E. H. (1969). 'Dissociated sensation in amyloidosis: compound action potential, quantitative histologic and teased-fiber, and electron microscopic studies of sural nerve biopsies.' *Arch. Neurol. (Chicago)*, **20**, 490.

Dyck, P. J. and Lambert, E. H. (1970). 'Polyneuropathy associated with hypothyroidism.' *J. Neuropath. Exp. Neurol.*, **29**, 631.

Dyck, P. J., Lambert, E. H. and Nichols, P. C. (1971b). 'Quantitative measurement of sensation related to compound action potential and number and sizes of myelinated and unmyelinated fibres of sural nerve in health, Friedreich's ataxia, hereditary sensory neuropathy and tabes dorsalis.' In *Handbook of Electroencephalography and Clinical Neurophysiology*, Vol. 9, p. 83. Amsterdam; Elsevier.

Eames, R. A. and Lange, L. S. (1967). 'Clinical and pathological study of ischaemic neuropathy.' *J. Neurol. Neurosurg. Psychiat.*, **20**, 215.

Emery, A. E. H. (1971). 'Review: the nosology of the spinal muscular atrophies.' *J. Med. Genet.*, **8**, 481.

Engel, A. G. and Santa, T. (1971). 'Histometric analysis of the ultrastructure of the neuromuscular junction in myasthenia gravis and in the myasthenic syndrome.' *Ann. N.Y. Acad. Sci.*, **183**, 46.

Erbslöh, F. and Abel, M. (1970). 'Deficiency neuropathies.' In *Handbook of Clinical Neurology*, Vol. 7. Ed. by P. J. Vinken and G. W. Bruyn. Amsterdam; North-Holland.

Esiri, M. M. and Tomlinson, A. H. (1972). 'Herpes zoster. Demonstration of virus in trigeminal nerve and ganglion by immunofluorescence and electron microscopy.' *J. Neurol. Sci.*, **15**, 35.

Fardeau, M. and Engel, W. K. (1969). 'Ultrastructural study of a peripheral nerve biopsy in Refsum's disease.' *J. Neuropath. Exp. Neurol.*, **28**, 278.

Finlayson, M. H., Bilbao, J. M. and Lough, J. O. (1974). 'The pathogenesis of the neuropathy in dimorphous leprosy: electron microscopic and cytochemical studies.' *J. Neuropath. Exp. Neurol.*, **33**, 446.

Fisher, C. M. and Adams, R. D. (1956). 'Diphtheritic paralysis: a pathological study.' *J. Neuropath. Exp. Neurol.*, **15**, 243.

Foster, J. B. (1974). 'The clinical features of some miscellaneous neuromuscular disorders.' In *Disorders of Voluntary Muscle*. Ed. by J. N. Walton. Edinburgh; Churchill Livingstone.

Franklin, E. C. (1974). 'The complexity of amyloid.' *New Engl. J. Med.*, **290**, 512.

Fullerton, P. M. (1966). 'Chronic peripheral neuropathy produced by lead poisoning in guinea-pigs.' *J. Neuropath. Exp. Neurol.*, **25**, 214.

Fullerton, P. M. and Barnes, J. M. (1966). 'Peripheral neuropathy in rats produced by acrylamide.' *Br. J. Indust. Med.*, **23**, 210.

Fullerton, P. M. and O'Sullivan, D. J. (1968). 'Thalidomide neuropathy: a clinical, electrophysiological and histological follow-up study.' *J. Neurol. Neurosurg. Pyschiat.*, **31**, 543.

Gardner-Medwin, D., Hudgson, P. and Walton, J. N. (1967). 'Benign spinal muscular atrophy arising in childhood and adolescence.' *J. Neurol. Sci.*, **5**, 121.

Garven, H. S. D., Gairns, F. W. and Smith, G. (1962). 'The nerve fibre populations of the leg in chronic occlusive arterial disease in man.' *Scot. Med. J.*, **7**, 250.

Gilliatt, R. W. (1973). 'Recent advances in the pathophysiology of nerve conduction.' In *New Developments in Electromyography and Clinical Electrophysiology*, Vol. 2, pp. 2–18. Ed. by J. E. Desmedt. Basle; Karger.

Glenner, G. C., Terry, W., Harada, M., Isersky, C. and Page, D. (1971). 'Amyloid fibril proteins: proof of homology with immunoglobulin light chains by sequence analysis.' *Science, N.Y.*, **172**, 1150.

Graham, J. G. and Oppenheimer, D. R. (1969). 'Orthostatic hypotension and nicotine sensitivity in a case of multiple system atrophy.' *J. Neurol. Neurosurg. Psychiat.*, **32**, 28.

REFERENCES

Grégoire, A., Perier, O. and Dustin, P. Jnr. (1966). 'Metachromatic leukodystrophy. An electron microscope study.' *J. Neuropath. Exp. Neurol.,* **25,** 617.

Gutmann, L. and Chou, S. M. (1976). 'Myasthenia gravis: current concepts.' *Arch. Pathol. Lab. Med.,* **100,** 401.

Hausmanowa-Petrusewicz, I. (1969). 'Infantile and juvenile spinal muscular atrophy.' In *Muscle Diseases. Proceedings International Congress, Milan, 1969.* Ed. by J. N. Walton, N. Canal and G. Scarlato. Amsterdam: Excerpta Medica.

Hayward, M. and Willison, R. G. (1973). 'The recognition of myogenic and neurogenic lesions by quantitative EMG.' In *New Developments in Electromyography and Clinical Neurophysiology,* Vol. 2, pp. 448–453. Ed. by J. E. Desmedt. Basle; Karger.

Heirons, R. (1957). 'Changes in the nervous system in acute porphyria.' *Brain,* **80,** 176.

Hensley, G. T. and Soergel, K. H. (1968). 'Neuropathologic findings in diabetic diarrhoea.' *Arch. Pathol.,* **85,** 587.

Henson, R. A. and Urich, H. (1970). 'Peripheral neuropathy associated with malignant disease.' *Handbook of Clinical Neurology,* Vol. 8, Ch. 9, p. 131. Ed. by P. J. Vinken and G. W. Bruyn. Amsterdam; North-Holland.

Hirano, A., Kurland, L. T. and Sayre, G. P. (1967). 'Familial amyotrophic lateral sclerosis.' *Arch. Neurol. (Chicago),* **16,** 232.

Hughes, J. T. (1966). In *Pathology of the Spinal Cord.* London; Lloyd-Luke.

Hughes, J. T., Brownell, B. and Hewer, R. L. (1968). 'The peripheral sensory pathway in Friedreich's ataxia. An examination by light and electron microscopy of posterior roots, posterior root ganglia and peripheral sensory nerves in a case of Friedreich's ataxia.' *Brain,* **91,** 803.

James, C. C. M. and Lassman, L. P. (1967). 'Results of treatment of progressive lesions in spina bifida occulta five to ten years after laminectomy.' *Lancet,* **ii,** 1277.

Job, C. K. (1973). 'Mechanisms of nerve destruction in tuberculoid borderline leprosy. An electron microscope study.' *J. Neurol. Sci.,* **20,** 25.

Johnson, R. H. and Spalding, J. M. K. (1974). In *Disorders of the Autonomic Nervous System.* Oxford; Blackwell.

Johnson, R. T. and Mims, C. A. (1968). 'Pathogenesis of viral infections of the nervous system.' *New Engl. J. Med.,* **278,** 23.

Johnson, R. T. and Richardson, E. P. (1968). 'The neurological manifestations of systemic lupus erythematosis.' *Medicine,* **47,** 333.

Joosten, E., Gabreëls, F., Gabréels-Festen, A., Vrensen, G., Korten, J. and Notermans, S. (1974). 'Electron-microscopic heterogeneity of onion-bulb neuropathies of the Dejerine–Sottas type.' *Acta Neuropath. (Berlin),* **27,** 105.

Kahn, P. (1973). 'Anderson–Fabry disease: a histopathological study of three cases with observations on the mechanisms of production of pain.' *J. Neurol. Neurosurg. Psychiat.,* **36,** 1056.

Kamensky, E., Philippart, M., Cancilla, P. and Frommes, S. P. (1973). 'Cultured skin fibroblasts in storage disorders. An analysis of ultrastructural features.' *Am. J. Pathol.,* **73,** 59.

Kashef, R. and Das Gupta, T. K. (1967). 'Segmental demyelination of peripheral nerves in the presence of malignant tumours.' *Br. J. Cancer,* **21,** 411.

Kibler, R. F. and Rose, F. C. (1960). 'Peripheral neuropathy in the "collagen diseases". A case of scleroderma neuropathy.' *Br. Med. J.,* **1,** 1781.

Klenk, A. and Kahlke, W. (1963). 'Uber das Vorkommen der 3.7.11. 15-Tetramethyl-hexadecan-saure (Phytansaure) in den Cholesterinestern und anderen Lipoidfraktionen der Organe bei einem Krankheitsfall unbekarmte, Genese (Verdacht auf Heredopathia atactica polyneuritiformis (Refsum-Syndrom)).' *Z. Physiol. Chem.,* **333,** 133.

Kocen, R. S., King, R. H. M., Thomas, P. K. and Haas, L. F. (1973). 'Nerve biopsy findings in two cases of Tangier disease.' *Acta Neuropath. (Berlin),* **26,** 317.

Kocen, R. S. and Thomas, P. K. (1970). 'Peripheral nerve involvement in Fabry's disease.' *Arch. Neurol. (Chicago),* **22,** 81.

Kristensson, K. and Olsson, Y. (1973). 'Diffusion pathways and retrograde axonal transport of protein tracers in peripheral nerves.' *Progr. Neurobiol.,* **1,** 85.

Lallemand, R. C. and Weller, R. O. (1973). 'Intraneural neurofibromas involving the posterior interosseous nerve.' *J. Neurol. Neurosurg. Psychiat.,* **36,** 991.

Lambert, E. H. and Dyck, P. J. (1968). 'Compound action potentials of human sural nerve biopsies.' *Electroenceph. Clin. Neurophysiol.,* **25,** 399.

Lampert, P. W. and Schochet, S. S. (1968). 'Demyelination and remyelination in lead neuropathy. Electron microscope studies.' *J. Neuropath. Exp. Neurol.,* **27,** 527.

141

REFERENCES

Lascelles, R. G. and Thomas, P. K. (1966). ' Changes due to age in internodal length in the sural nerve in man.' *J. Neurol. Neurosurg. Psychiat.*, **29,** 40.

Lee, R. G. and White, D. G. (1973). 'Computer analysis of motor unit action potentials in routine clinical electromyography.' In *New Developments in Electromyography and Clinical Neurophysiology,* Vol. 2, pp. 454–461. Ed. by J. E. Desmedt. Basle; Karger.

Lever, W. F. (1967). In *Histopathology of the Skin,* 4th edn. Philadelphia; Lippincott.

Liu, H. M. (1968). 'Ultrastructure of central nervous system lesions in metachromatic leukodystrophy with special reference to morphogenesis.' *J. Neuropath. Exp. Neurol.,* **27,** 624.

Liversedge, L. A. and Campbell, M. J. (1974). 'The central neuronal muscular atrophies and other dysfunctions of the anterior horn cells.' In *Disorders of Voluntary Muscle,* p. 775. Ed. by J. N. Walton. Edinburgh; Churchill Livingstone.

Lyon, G. (1969). 'Ultrastructural study of a nerve biopsy from a case of early infantile chronic neuropathy.' *Acta Neuropath. (Berlin),* **13,** 131.

McLeod, J. G. (1971). 'An electrophysiological and pathological study of peripheral nerves in Friedreich's ataxia.' *J. Neurol. Sci.,* **12,** 333.

McLeod, J. C., Walsh, J. C. and Little, J. M. (1969). 'Sural nerve biopsy.' *Med. J. Australia,* **II,** 1092.

Manson-Bahr, P. (1966). In *Manson's Tropical Diseases,* 16th edn. London; Baillière, Tindall and Cassell.

Mars, H., Lewis, L. A., Robertson, A. L., Butkus, A. and Williams, G. H. (1969). 'Familial hypo-β-lipoproteinemia.' *Am. J. Med.,* **46,** 886.

Matthews, W. B. (1965). 'Sarcoidosis of the nervous system.' *J. Neurol. Neurosurg. Psychiat.,* **28,** 23.

Milhorat, T. H. (1972). In *Hydrocephalus and the Cerebrospinal Fluid.* Baltimore; Williams and Wilkins.

Neary, D. and Eames, R. A. (1975). 'The pathology of ulnar nerve compression in man.' *Neuropathol. Appl. Neurobiol.,* **1,** 69.

O'Brien, M. D. (1968). 'Hypertrophic neuropathy: A report of Dejerine–Sottas disease in two sibs.' *Guy's Hosp. Rept.,* **117,** 79.

Ochoa, J. (1970). 'Isoniazid neuropathy in man: quantitative electron microscope study.' *Brain,* **93,** 831.

Ochoa, J., Danta, G., Fowler, T. J. and Gilliatt, R. W. (1971). 'Nature of the nerve lesion caused by a pneumatic tourniquet.' *Nature (London),* **233,** 265.

Ochoa, J. and Mair, W. G. P. (1969). 'The normal sural nerve in man. II. Changes in the axons and Schwann cells due to ageing.' *Acta Neuropath. (Berlin),* **13,** 217.

Ohta, M., Ellefson, R. D., Lambert, E. H. and Dyck, P. J. (1973). 'Hereditary sensory neuropathy, Type 2. Clinical electrophysiologic, histologic and biochemical studies of a Quebec kinship.' *Arch. Neurol. (Chicago),* **29,** 23.

Pearn, J. H., Carter, C. O. and Wilson, J. (1973). 'The genetic identity of acute infantile spinal muscular atrophy.' *Brain,* **96,** 463.

Pearse, A. G. E. (1968). In *Histochemistry—Theoretical and Applied,* 3rd edn, Vol. 1. London; Churchill.

Pollard, J. D., McLeod, J. G. and Gye, R. S. (1973). 'Regeneration through peripheral nerve allografts.' *Arch. Neurol. (Chicago),* **28,** 31.

Pratt, R. T. C. (1967). In *The Genetics of Neurological Disorders.* London; University Press.

Prineas, J. (1969a). 'The pathogenesis of dying-back neuropathies. Part I. An ultrastructural study of experimental tri-ortho-cresyl phosphate poisoning.' *J. Neuropath. Exp. Neurol.,* **28,** 571.

Prineas, J. (1969b). 'The pathogenesis of dying-back neuropathies. Part 2. An ultrastructural study of experimental acrylamide intoxication in the rat.' *J. Neuropath. Exp. Neurol.,* **28,** 598.

Prineas, J. W. (1970). 'Polyneuropathies of undetermined cause.' *Acta Neurol. Scand.,* **46,** Suppl. 44, 3.

Prineas, J. W. (1972). 'Acute idiopathic polyneuritis: an electron microscope study.' *Lab. Invest.,* **26,** 133.

Raff, M. C. and Asbury, A. K. (1968). 'Ischemic mononeuropathy and mononeuropathy multiplex in diabetes mellitus.' *New Engl. J. Med.,* **279,** 17.

Rees, R. J. W. and Waters, M. F. R. (1971). 'Recent trends in leprosy research.' *Br. Med. Bull.,* **12,** 16.

Ridley, A. (1969). 'The neuropathy of acute intermittent porphyria.' *Quart. J. Med.,* **38,** 307.

Ridley, D. S. (1973). 'The pathogenesis of the early skin lesions in leprosy.' *J. Pathol.,* **111,** 191.
142

REFERENCES

Russell, D. S. (1953). 'Histological changes in the striped muscles in myasthenia gravis.' *J. Pathol. Bacteriol.*, **65**, 279.

Schaumburg, H. H., Wisniewski, H. M. and Spencer, P. S. (1974). 'Ultrastructural studies of the dying-back process. I. Peripheral nerve terminal and axonal degeneration in systemic acrylamide intoxication.' *J. Neuropath. Exp. Neurol.*, **33**, 260.

Schoene, W. C., Asbury, A. K., Aström, K. E. and Masters, R. (1970). 'Hereditary sensory neuropathy. A clinical and ultrastructural study.' *J. Neurol. Sci.*, **11**, 463.

Schwartz, J. F., Rowland, L. P., Eder, H., Marks, P. A., Osserman, E. F., Hirschberg, E. and Anderson, H. (1963). 'Bassen−Kornzweig syndrome: deficiency of serum β-lipoprotein.' *Arch. Neurol. (Chicago)*, **8**, 438.

Siggers, D. (1975). Personal communication.

Simpson, J. A. (1974). 'Myasthenia gravis and myasthenic syndromes.' In *Disorders of Voluntary Muscle*. Ed. by J. N. Walton. Edinburgh; Churchill Livingstone.

Smith, B. (1970). 'Disorders of the myenteric plexus.' *Gut*, **11**, 271.

Sourander, P. and Olsson, Y. (1968). 'Peripheral neuropathy in globoid cell leucodystrophy (Morbus Krabbe).' *Acta Neuropath. (Berlin)*, **11**, 69.

Steinberg, D., Mize, C. E., Herndon, J. H., Fales, H. M., Engel, W. K. and Vroom, F. Q. (1970). 'Phytanic acid in patients with Refsum's syndrome and response to dietary treatment.' *Arch. Intern. Med.*, **66**, 365.

Steinberg, D., Vroom, F. Q., Engel, K. W., Cammermeyer, J., Mize, C. E. and Avigan, J. (1967). 'Refsum's disease. A recently characterized lipidosis involving the nervous system.' *Arch. Intern Med.*, **66**, 365.

Stewart, C. R. and Ward, A. M. (1974). 'Experiences in the clinical management of amniotic alpha-fetoprotein estimations.' *Develop. Med. Child Neurol.*, **16**, Suppl. 32, 126.

Sunderland, S. (1968). In *Nerve and Nerve Injuries*. Edinburgh; Livingstone.

Symonds, C. P. and Blackwood, W. (1962). 'Spinal cord compression in hypertrophic neuritis.' *Brain*, **85**, 251.

Thomas, P. K. (1973). 'The ultrastructural pathology of unmyelinated nerve fibres.' In *New Developments in Electromyography and Clinical Neurophysiology*, Vol. 2, p. 227. Ed. by J. E. Desmedt. Basle; Karger.

Thomas, P. K., Hollinrake, K., Lascelles, R. G., O'Sullivan, D. J., Baillod, R. A., Moorhead, J. F. and MacKenzie, J. C. (1971). 'The polyneuropathy of chronic renal failure.' *Brain*, **94**, 761.

Thomas, P. K. and Lascelles, R. G. (1966). 'The pathology of diabetic neuropathy.' *Quart. J. Med.*, **35**, 489.

Thomas, P. K., Lascelles, R. G., Hallpike, J. F. and Hewer, R. L. (1969). 'Recurrent and chronic relapsing Guillain−Barré polyneuritis.' *Brain*, **92**, 589.

Thomashefsky, A. J., Horwitz, S. J. and Feingold, M. H. (1972). 'Acute autonomic neuropathy.' *Neurology*, **22**, 251.

Vinken, P. J. and Bruyn, G. W. (Editors) (1970). *Handbook of Clinical Neurology*, Vols. 7, 8: *Diseases of Nerves*. Amsterdam; North-Holland.

Walton, J. N. (1968). 'Classification of the neuromuscular disorders.' *J. Neurol. Sci.*, **6**, 165.

Warrell, D. A., Godfrey, S. and Olsen, E. G. J. (1968). 'Giant-cell arteritis with peripheral neuropathy.' *Lancet*, **i**, 1010.

Weller, R. O. (1967). 'An electron microscope study of hypertrophic neuropathy of Dejerine−Sottas.' *J. Neurol. Neurosurg. Psychiat.*, **30**, 111.

Weller, R. O., Bruckner, F. E. and Chamberlain, M. A. (1970). 'Rheumatoid neuropathy: a histological and electrophysiological study.' *J. Neurol. Neurosurg. Psychiat.*, **33**, 592.

Widerholt, W. C., Mulder, D. W. and Lambert, E. H. (1964). 'The Landry−Guillain−Barré−Strohl syndrome or polyradiculoneuropathy: historical review, report on 97 patients and present concepts.' *Mayo Clin. Proc.*, **30**, 427.

Williams, B. and Weller, R. O. (1973). 'Syringomyelia produced by intramedullary fluid injection in dogs.' *J. Neurol. Neurosurg. Psychiat.*, **36**, 467.

Willis, R. A. (1962). In *The Borderland of Embryology and Pathology*, 2nd edn. London; Butterworths.

Wisniewski, H., Terry, R. D., Whitaker, J. N., Cook, S. D. and Dowling, P. C. (1969). 'Landry−Guillain−Barré syndrome: a primary demyelinating disease.' *Arch. Neurol. (Chicago)*, **21**, 269.

Woolf, A. L. (1966). 'Morphology of the myasthenic neuromuscular junction.' *Ann. N.Y. Acad. Sci.*, **135**, Art. 1, 35.

Yoshizumi, M. O. and Asbury, A. K. (1974). 'Intra-axonal bacilli in lepromatous leprosy: a light and electron microscopic study.' *Acta Neuropath. (Berlin)*, **27**, 1.

Young, J. Z. (1942). 'Functional repair of nervous tissue.' *Physiol. Rev.*, **22**, 318.

6

Tumours of the Peripheral Nervous System

The majority of tumours in the peripheral nervous system are derived from Schwann cells and other peripheral nerve elements. They arise mainly in cranial and spinal nerves and their roots, but similar tumours also occur in the peripheral autonomic nervous system. Neoplasms of the peripheral nervous system originating from nerve cells or their processes, on the other hand, are almost entirely confined to the autonomic nervous system; they include tumours of adrenal medulla and other sites in the chromaffin system.

In oncology, more than in other fields of pathology, individual schools are unable to arrive at a common agreement on terminology. The terminology used in this chapter is that recommended by the *Committee of Tumour Nomenclature and Statistics of the International Union Against Cancer, 'Unio Internationalis Contra Cancrum' (UICC)* (Springer, Berlin–Heidelberg–New York, 1965) in so far as the lesions are included in their classification. Exceptions have been made in cases where the terms proposed in the classification are obviously misleading or have not yet been substantiated by the newer techniques. The UICC classification is pragmatic, utilizing the frequently used and well-recognized names even though they may no longer be scientifically correct. As many pathologists and most clinicians may not be familiar with the classification, the common synonyms for each tumour will be mentioned.

Table 4 summarizes the neoplasms and the tumour-like non-neoplastic lesions that can occur in the peripheral nervous system. In this chapter only the tumour entities of major importance will be treated *in extenso*; in *Table 4* these lesions are in italics. Rarer tumours are briefly described with their relevant bibliography. Multiple neurofibromatosis (von Recklinghausen's disease) will not be treated as a complete entity, since the changes are neither restricted to the peripheral nervous system nor to the nervous system as a whole. However, the peripheral nerve tumours occurring in neurofibromatosis are dealt with in the different sections of this chapter, especially in the section devoted to neurofibromas. Electron microscopy has led to the most important advances in the field of peripheral nerve tumours in the last 20 years.

Therefore, despite the small number of publications that deal with the ultrastructure of these tumours, and some contradictory interpretation of the results, special emphasis will be placed upon the electron microscopic findings if they are available. The recent works of Harkin and Reed (1968) and Krücke (1974) are recommended for their excellent and extensive histological descriptions and illustrations.

TABLE 4

A. Non-neoplastic tumour- like growths	*Traumatic neuroma* Plantar neuroma Localized hypertrophic neuropathy Perivascular Schwannosis Pseudocysts of the nerve
B. Tumours of the nerve sheath	*Neurinoma* Granular cell neurinoma *Neurofibroma* Multiple mucosal neuroma *Malignant tumours*
C. Tumours of nerve cell origin	*Neuroblastoma* Ganglioneuroma
D. Tumours of non-nervous origin	Pheochromocytoma

A. NON-NEOPLASTIC TUMOUR-LIKE GROWTHS

TRAUMATIC NEUROMA

Synonyms: Pseudoneuroma; amputation neuroma; hyperplastic scar of the nerve.

Incidence, location and clinical data

Whenever a nerve is severed, anywhere in the body, a scar forms at the site of nerve section. The scar may be quite small and only the large or symptomatic lesions are termed traumatic neuromas; this explains the occasional statement that in some cases the amputation of a nerve is not followed by the formation of a neuroma. Traumatic neuromas can also follow a nerve crush where the continuity between proximal and distal segments is retained. Neuromas are tender and sensitive to pressure. Pain may be referred to the area normally innervated by the severed nerve, but correlation of the so-called 'phantom limb' phenomenon with the presence of a traumatic neuroma is not usually possible. Why some neuromas are painful whereas others of the same size, or even larger, are free of pain remains unexplained. One theory is that the pain-conducting C-fibres are more resistant to ischaemia, so that only they, of all the neural elements, survive in the relatively avascular neuroma. Visceral neuromas following surgical procedures have been described after gastrectomy, cholecystectomy and nephrectomy; they are often asymptomatic.

The tendency to overlook neuromas prevails when they occur in sites other than amputation sites. Lack of a definite pattern of symptoms produced by such lesions is probably the most important reason for this oversight (Mathews and Osterholm, 1972).

In sites such as the hands, feet and face, where minor injuries are common, typical traumatic neuromas may be identified histologically even though the patient may not remember the injury (Harkin and Reed, 1969).

Gross appearance

Transection of a nerve produces a terminal neuroma, whereas a partial injury causes an eccentric nodular appendage to develop on the injured side of the nerve. Repeated blunt trauma results in a fusiform swelling of the nerve trunk termed a neuroma-in-continuity. Grossly, they are firm, irregular oval nodules varying in size, but rarely larger than a pea. The outer layer of fibrous tissue is often inseparable from the surrounding scar, and the avascular nature of the neuroma is suggested by the white fibrous appearance of the cut surface.

Microscopic appearances

Traumatic neuromas are composed of axons, Schwann cells, endoneurial cells and perineurial cells in a dense collagenous matrix. In the early stages, some 3–6 months following trauma, the end of the nerve is oedematous and contains a large amount of mucinous matrix. Varying numbers of non-

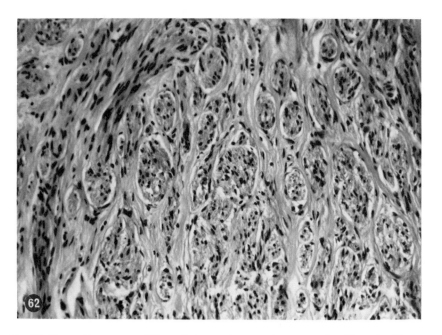

Fig. 62. Traumatic neuroma of the radial nerve 4 years after amputation. Nerve fascicles are surrounded by a dense collagenous stroma. H. and E. stain; ×120

myelinated and myelinated axons form a tangle of nerve fibres separated into compact tiny fascicles. Many Schwann cell cords within the fascicles are associated with axons, but some contain no axons at all. Layers of perineurium form around each fascicle and the adjacent tissue is converted into dense fibrous tissue (*Figure 62*). In the late stages much of the neuroma may consist of collagen.

Electron microscopic appearances

The ultrastructural appearance of a traumatic neuroma varies widely, depending upon the area explored; the constituent elements, however, are fairly constant. Nerve fibres near the proximal nerve trunk are often myelinated (*Figure 63*), but in the distal zones myelinated axons are rare or non-existent. There is a predominance of thin unmyelinated axons when compared with a normal nerve, and a variety of different axon–Schwann cell relationships are seen. In addition to the usual invagination of the axon by the Schwann cell, with the formation of regular mesaxons, some axons are situated at the surface of the Schwann cell and separated from the interstitial space only by the basement membrane. Occasionally a whole group of axons is seen surrounded by a Schwann cell but without Schwann cytoplasm separating the individual fibres. With increasing fibrosis, the Schwann cells ensheath bundles of collagen fibres and axons become rare (*Figure 64*).

Elongated cell processes are also seen (*Figure 63*); some of these cells are

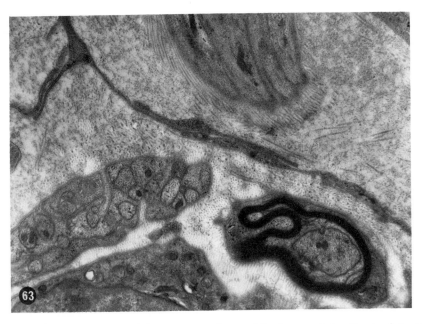

Fig. 63. Traumatic neuroma of the sciatic nerve 9 years following amputation. Proximal stump of the nerve showing myelinated and non-myelinated nerve fibres embedded in a dense fibrous stroma. In the centre of the field, elongated cell processes are in loose contact with each other. Electron micrograph ×9000

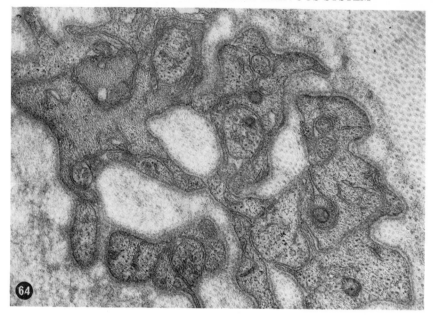

Fig. 64. *The same traumatic neuroma as in Figure 63 but in the distal stump of the nerve. Note the increase in the number of collagen fibres and the collagen pockets formed by the Schwann cells. Electron micrograph ×20 000*

surrounded by basement membrane which suggests a perineurial or Schwann cell origin. The majority of these cells, however, have no basement membrane and are probably derived from endoneurial fibroblasts. The thin cell processes interdigitate, but they seldom form true junctional complexes. In many cases the cells and their processes surround bundles of nerve fibres and Schwann cells, and occasionally they are arranged in layers like onion-bulbs. Some of the cell processes are also in a loose arrangement and have no definite relationship either to axons or to their Schwann cells.

The interstitial space is more extensive in the distal parts of a neuroma, but as yet the oedematous areas of mucinous matrix in early neuromas have not been studied ultrastructurally; this is mainly because only chronic neuromas are usually explored surgically, and by this time the main component of the interstitial space is collagen. Multilayered basement membranes and cross-striated fibrillary bundles (see *Figures 79* and *80*) were seldom seen in our cases, but they have been described in other ultrastructural studies of traumatic neuromas (Hilding and House, 1965; Poirier and Escourolle, 1970).

Pathogenesis and differential diagnosis

Newly formed nerve sprouts grow out from the proximal end of a severed nerve into the distal segment: a phenomenon which involves 'neurobiotaxis'. Vigorous growth of axon sprouts begins within the proximal stump of the nerve during the first 2–3 days, and the nerve sprouts, together with their supporting Schwann cells, can produce the unmistakable histological appearance of a neuroma within 3 weeks (Huber and Lewis, 1920). The proximal stump acquires a cap of fibroblasts and a scar quickly forms; all but a few of the regenerating axons find this barrier impenetrable. Schwann cells lose their orientation and the axons turn back on themselves and grow in a retrograde manner for short distances, assuming the irregular spiral appearance initially described by Perroncito (1907). Short processes known as growth cones form and represent abortive attempts at branching. Axons that cross the defect in the nerve appear to influence the direction of growth of adjacent axons, so that closely bunched groups of fascicles are formed. Proliferation of the axons and Schwann cells is probably halted eventually because of crowding and because the meagre blood supply is soon outstripped. Fibres that escape the connective tissue cap have been shown to wander over long distances into surrounding tissue along fascial planes and along blood vessels; these axons are thought by many to be more responsible for pain than the neuroma itself. Although the circuituous route taken by the axons is usually attributed to the presence of an obstacle, an alternative possibility is that the matrix of the perineurium has a trophic influence upon the axons. Myelination keeps pace with the growth of the axons both inside and outside the neuroma.

Once formed, little change seems to occur within the neuroma. Maturation of the connective tissue cap, some loss of neural elements and a relative increase in the Schwann cell population occur, lending credence to the concept of sclerosing neuromata.

If clinical data do not point to the traumatic origin, a traumatic neuroma can be mistaken for a neurofibroma; this is understandable because the same growth factor is probably responsible for the two lesions. In traumatic neuromas this factor acts locally and only once, i.e. as a consequence of loss of continuity of the nerve. In neurofibromatosis, however, the growth factor acts throughout life and at different sites as a consequence of a genetic disturbance (p. 177). Histologically, the differentiation of multiple mucosal neuromas from traumatic neuromas, which they resemble, can be difficult. The localization and gross appearance of these lesions, however, makes the differential diagnosis much easier.

The onion-bulbs seen in a Morton's neuroma (see below; Webster, Schröder, Asbury and Adams, 1967) are much larger than the onion-bulb whorls of hypertrophic neuropathy (see pp. 83 et seq.), and the two lesions can hardly be confused.

Plantar neuroma

Synonyms: Morton's neuroma; nodular interdigital nerve scar; localizing interdigital neuritis; sclerosing neuroma.

Localized degeneration and proliferative reaction in one or more of the interdigital plantar nerves can occur with the formation of a swelling near the heads of the metatarsal bones. The disease is more common in women and possibly relates to the design of their shoes, which often compress the metatarsal heads. Ninety per cent of cases involve the nerves of the second and third clefts, followed in order of frequency by the nerves in the fourth and fifth clefts (Graham and Johnston, 1957). The chief symptom is chronic pain, which is only occasionally severe but may radiate into the leg or may present as tingling and numbness in the distribution of the nerve. Pain may be paroxysmal, and has been compared with that associated with peripheral arterial insufficiency.

Macroscopically, the nerve is thickened in the area of involvement and expanded to form a grey, pale nodule less than 1 cm in diameter. The lesion is circumscribed but not encapsulated and is adherent to the adjacent artery and synovial sheath of the intermetatarsal bursa. Histologically, there is degeneration of axons and myelin in the area of involvement. Extracellular collagen and mucinous matrix in the perineurium and epineurium is markedly increased. Rounded nodules or onion-bulbs are prominent in some lesions; these are composed of concentric lamellae formed from bundles of collagen and they are devoid of cells. The small arteries are usually thickened and may contain thrombi (Nissen, 1951).

The aetiology of the plantar neuroma is not known, but degeneration of the nerve may be caused by trauma and is probably the result of repeated minor insults which damage the arteries associated with the nerve as well as the nerve itself. Scarring of the posterior interosseous nerve adjacent to the fibula may occasionally resemble Morton's neuroma. Although probably caused by trauma, Morton's neuromas differ from amputation or traumatic neuromas, which are composed of numerous intertwined small nerve fascicles or nerve fibres with a disrupted perineurium.

LOCALIZED 'HYPERTROPHIC NEUROPATHY'

Synonyms: Intraneural neurofibroma; fibroma; fibrous lesion of the nerve.

Local nerve swellings similar to those of the plantar nerves of the foot may arise in the median nerve at the wrist and in the ulnar nerve at the elbow. They are often accompanied by overt nerve fibre damage, and thus easily recognized clinically (Ochoa and Neary, 1975). These lesions are universally regarded as the consequence of repeated trauma. Similar swellings are fairly consistently found in relatively inconspicuous nerves such as the dorsal interosseous branch of the radial nerve as it passes over the back of the wrist; the terminal portion of the lateral branch of the deep peroneal nerve; and the posterior branch of the axillary nerve supplying the teres minor muscle (Daniell, 1954). Such minor enlargements are usually in close contact with tendons, ligaments, muscle or bone. In view of the predictable absence of ganglion cells and the degree of focal fibrosis, it has been quite justifiably proposed that these lesions are acquired as a result of friction and chronic trauma in a similar way to the major entrapment lesions (Gitlin, 1957).

Lallemend and Weller (1973) have drawn special attention to the lesions of the posterior interosseous nerve and they have studied them electron microscopically. The true incidence of these lesions is not known, as many of the reported cases have not been explored surgically. Clinically, there is a posterior interosseous nerve palsy with supinator weakness without sensory disturbance or pain. The nerve swelling is localized proximal to the supinator

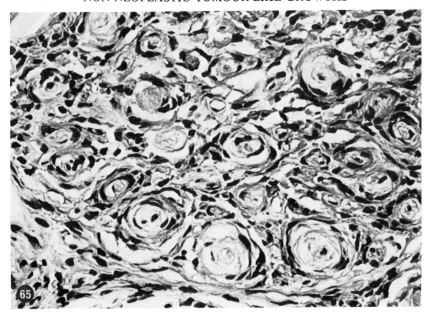

Fig. 65 Localized hypertrophy of the posterior interosseous nerve in a 20 year old woman. Transverse section of the swollen nerve fascicle showing cellular whorls up to 50 µm in diameter. H. and E. stain; ×430 *(Courtesy of Lallemand and Weller, 1973, and* J. Neurol. Neurosurg. Psychiat.*)*

tunnel. Histologically, the lesions display a whorl-like pattern that has previously been confused with the onion-bulb structures in hypertrophic polyneuropathy (Weller, 1974; *Figure 65*); there is an almost total loss of myelinated fibres and a moderate increase in cellularity. Thickening and fibrosis of the endoneurial septa and the perineurium is seen, and the endoneurial collagen is also increased. No inflammatory cells have been observed and the vessels appear normal. Electron microscopically, the cells forming the whorls differ in several ways from normal human Schwann cells, and the ring-shaped structures seen in transverse sections of the nerve are often formed by several cells. The basement membrane is incomplete around these cells; their processes interdigitate and frequently form junctional complexes. The centre of the cellular ring is occupied by collagen and fragments of amorphous material; some of the collagen bundles are orientated circumferentially. In addition to the whorls, the abnormal cells may be seen in compact groups sometimes around blood vessels. Those Schwann cells associated with normal axons, or with the occasional axon balloon, appear normal. Scattered fibroblasts were seen in the lesion and can be distinguished from the cells forming the ring-shaped structures.

There are several features that are against trauma being directly responsible: the onset of the paresis is usually slow; the nerve lesions in both cases were proximal to the usual site of compression by the supinator muscle; and the histology does not resemble that of a traumatic neuroma. Therefore, Lallemand and Weller (1973) favoured a neoplastic nature and regarded them as neurofibromas. Nevertheless, they pointed to the fact that no other stigmata of von Recklinghausen's disease have been seen in the reported cases and asked the question why neurofibromata should arise in this particular site on the posterior interosseous nerve. Since localized neural hypertrophy at different sites closely resembles plantar neuromas, a similar pathogenic mechanism should be postulated for all these lesions, and a traumatic origin seems at present the most probable.

Perivascular Schwannosis

Synonyms: Spinal neuroma; aberrant regenerating nerve fibres; hyperplasia of nerve elements.

Nerves running in the adventitia of the vessels of the spinal cord and of the meninges can proliferate to form small nodules (*Figure 66*). These peculiar lesions were first reported by Raymond in 1893 and have since been seen by a considerable number of authors and attributed to a wide variety of causes. Allowing for a slight degree of variation among these authors, the appearance and light microscopy of these proliferations is as follows: they are almost always located in perivascular areas (and/or in the vicinity of the posterior roots) and are more or less clearly defined from the surrounding tissue; confluent nodules or fascicles of intermingling whorls of spindle-shaped cells are found. The cells are slender, with elongated nuclei and scant polar cytoplasm. Nuclear palisading is not conspicuous, and Verocay bodies, areas of necrosis and microcystic degeneration are not seen. Among the interlacing cells, structures resembling

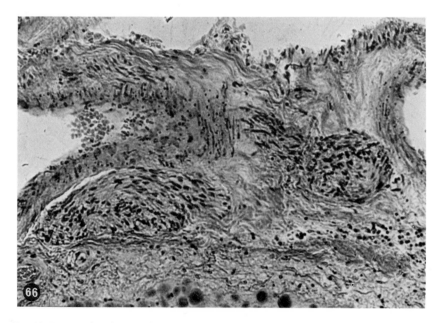

Fig. 66. Perivascular clusters of cells (Schwannosis) in the meninges of the spinal cord in a 94 year old man. H. and E. stain; ×270

myelinated nerve fibres, but staining atypically with myelin stains, are seen with varying frequency.

From a morphological point of view, the cellular proliferations fall into two types, although biologically they are probably identical. First, there are nodules which are mostly globoid in shape and range up to several millimetres in diameter; these are infrequent but can produce clinical signs. Second, discrete groups of cells, sometimes as few as ten in number, are often seen typically arranged as perivascular whorls. Staemmler (1939) found such groups in 26 out of 600 cases, Riggs and Clary (1957) in 14 of 36 cases and Ferszt (1974) in 7 of 27 cases. The small groups of cells are usually spread throughout the entire cord and, although not limited to these areas, they are certainly seen most often in the perivascular areas of the sulcocommissural arteries and near the posterior roots. It is an interesting point that the tendency to produce these structures varies from case to case. They are rarely solitary, but, rather, the inherent capacity to produce them leads to multiplicity. Hori (1973) consequently chose the term 'Schwannosis' to characterize these structures, stressing their diffuse nature.

Ultrastructurally (Bernstein, Collins and Bernstein, 1973; Ferszt, 1974), at least two cell types are easily discernible: (1) slender fibrocyte-like cells which are loosely interlacing and embedded in a large amount of homogeneous intercellular substance and strands of collagen; (2) myelinated nerve fibres with Schmidt–Lantermann incisures.

It is thus apparent that these lesions are neurofibromatous, but their origin remains an enigma. Attempts to correlate the structures with a specific disease have not been entirely successful. They have been reported in syringomyelia, trauma, prolapsed intervertebral discs, tabes, Pott's disease, myeloma and multiple neurofibromatosis (Beck, 1939; Staemmler, 1939; Riggs and Clary, 1959), and with advanced age. It seems that they have been seen in almost every instance where the tissue has been meticulously studied. At the present time it is reasonable to conclude that the proliferation of perivascular nerves in the spinal cord and meninges is a relatively non-specific reaction to a variety of stimuli. Such a reaction could well occur in a considerable percentage of the population. The pathogenetic mechanism underlying these changes, and their possible relationship to a latent form of neurofibromatosis, are, as yet, poorly understood.

Interfascicular pseudocysts of nerves

Synonyms: Mucinous ganglion cyst; ganglion of the peroneal nerve; myxofibroma; arthroma.

Mucin-filled cysts have been reported, mainly involving the peroneal nerve in the vicinity of the knee joint (Barrett and Cramer, 1963). They have no epithelial lining and are therefore not true cysts. Pseudocysts involving the radial nerve at the wrist have also been reported (Harkin and Reed, 1969). They tend to recur and the end-stage may be total interruption of the nerve.

Reviewing 67 cases in the literature, Krücke (1974) found that compression of the nerve in 34 cases was a consequence of an extraneural pseudocyst, and in 33 cases, of an intraneural pseudocyst. The gross appearance of the mucin-

153

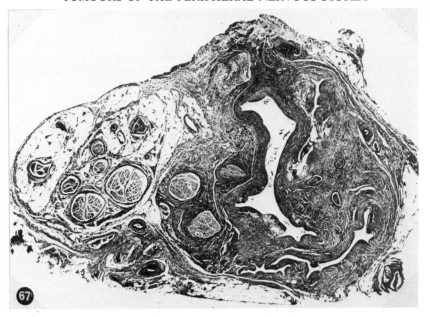

Fig. 67. Transverse section through the peroneal nerve of a 61 year old man. Four pseudocysts are seen with dense fibrosis of the epineurial tissue and shrinkage of the nerve fascicles. At the top of the picture, normal epineurium surrounds normal nerve fascicles. (Courtesy of W. Krücke, Pathologie der peripheren Nerven. Hdb. der Neurochirurgie, *Vol. VII/3; Springer, Berlin)*

filled cyst is characteristic. Occasionally it can be mistaken for a cystic neurinoma, which in some cases may reach a large size. In contrast to the cystic neurinoma, however, the wall of the pseudocyst is compact and white in colour; it is formed mainly of collagen. Occasionally there is some lining by endothelial-like cells but with no epithelial component (*Figure 67*). Circumscribed areas of myxomatous change and foam-cell accumulation are sometimes seen in the subcapsular regions. The histological appearances are the same whether the cyst is in the epineurium between fascicles or in the endoneurium within a nerve fascicle (Krücke, 1974). Therefore, it is unlikely that the pseudocysts result from the degeneration within a neural tumour. Their location at points of mechanical stress favours a traumatic aetiology; this would also account for the frequent occurrence of pseudocysts in relation to joints.

B. TUMOURS OF THE NERVE SHEATH

The histogenesis and nomenclature of these neoplasms remain a matter of much debate but essentially revolve around two issues. The first concerns the cell of origin, for which two candidates have long been proposed: the Schwann cell (Verocay, 1908; Antoni, 1920), on the one hand, and the fibroblast (Penfield, 1932), on the other.

Some authors consider that neurinomas originate from perineurial cells, but they do not agree upon the origin of this cell. Tarlov (1940), Waggener (1966), Poirier and Escourolle (1967) and Raimondo and Beckman (1967) think that perineurial cells have a fibroblastic origin, whereas others feel that they are derived from Schwann cells (Masson, 1942; Harkin and Reed, 1968). Inherent to this aspect of the controversy is the presence of collagen and reticulin fibres in these tumours and the question of whether the Schwann cell, as well as the fibroblast, is capable of synthesizing collagen. The second point of discussion is whether the nerve sheath tumours constitute a single entity or whether they should be divided into two separate morphological groups: namely, neurinomas, on the one hand, and neurofibromas, on the other.

Although the advent of the electron microscope has initially complicated rather than simplified the problem (Rubinstein, 1972), the ultrastructural findings available at the present time have given us a better insight into these problems. The problems of histogenesis and nomenclature, therefore, will be discussed after the electron microscope findings have been described. For the moment the distinction between neurinoma and neurofibroma will be maintained. This distinction has clinical implications, since neurinomas seldom recur, whereas recurrence and malignant change are found among the neurofibromas.

NEURINOMA

Synonyms: Solitary Schwannoma; neurilemoma; perineurial fibroblastoma; acoustic neuroma.

Incidence, location and clinical data

Neurinomas occur in every part of the peripheral nervous system but are most commonly found on the sensory cranial nerves and the sensory posterior spinal roots. The intracranial portion of the acoustic nerve is the site of more than 60 per cent of all neurinomas (*Figure 68*). They represent one-third of the tumours in the posterior fossa (Cervós-Navarro, 1969) and about 8 per cent of all intracranial tumours. The rest of the cranial nerves are seldom the site of solitary neurinomas except for the trigeminal nerve and the Gasserian ganglion where they occasionally occur. Neurinomas of the spinal nerve roots (*Figure 69* and *70*) represent about one-fourth of spinal tumours; they may be situated either within or outside the dura, intra- or extravertebral, or a combination of both with a narrow attachment through the intervertebral foramen (dumb-bell tumour). Every major peripheral nerve can be the site of a neurinoma, but tumours of the fine nerves in the subcutaneous tissue and skin are almost exclusively neurofibromas; if neurinomas are described in this location, the accuracy of the diagnosis is questionable (Harkin and Reed, 1968). Multiple neurinomas with exactly the same histological pattern as that of the solitary tumours are frequently found in neurofibromatosis, but seldom occur unassociated with this syndrome (Krücke, 1974).

Neurinomas have been described at various sites in the sympathetic nervous system, and less often on the vagus nerve (Sarin, Bennett and Jackson, 1974). In both these sites, however, the tumours are mostly neurofibromas. The large

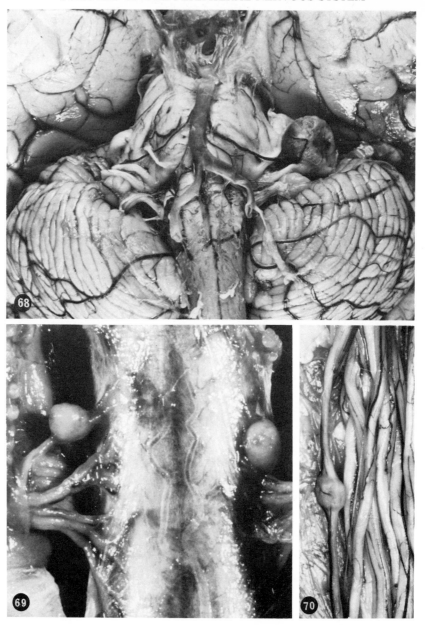

Fig. 68. Neurinoma of the left eighth cranial nerve (acoustic neurinoma). The nerve of origin is compressed at the periphery of the tumour

Fig. 69. Multiple neurinomas in the motor roots of C_1 and C_2 in a 68 year old man with no signs of neurofibromatosis

Fig. 70. Neurinoma in a sensory root of the caudal equina. Incidental finding in a 49 year old woman

majority of reports are of coincidental findings of nodules ranging from the size of 'hemp seed' to 'cherry stone' and occurring in the intestinal tract. They have seldom been clinically diagnosed, but occasionally they reach a considerable size.

Neurinomas occur approximately twice as frequently in women as in men. There is no obvious predilection for any ethnic group and the incidence is greatest in the middle decades (mean age, 40 years). Depending upon their location and size, neurinomas may produce a large variety of symptoms, but they are usually asymptomatic when small. Furthermore the slow rate of growth of neurinomas allows surrounding structures to adapt to the tumour's expansion, and asymptomatic neurinomas, therefore, are frequently an incidental finding at autopsy. The earliest and most striking symptoms in acoustic neurinoma are auditory, in the form of tinnitus and progressive loss of hearing. Vestibular involvement is less severe, and generally consists of either subjective or objective vertigo. Except for damage to the homolateral seventh nerve, involvement of other cranial nerves is often variable and, in many cases, inconstant. Compression of the adjacent cerebellar hemispheres or the cerebellar peduncles results in ataxia, vertigo and other evidence of cerebellar dysfunction.

Because of their preference for the posterior spinal roots, the first symptoms of intraspinal neurinomas are sensory. Motor symptoms develop if the tumour compresses the anterior roots. Neurinomas in the more peripheral parts of the nerve may cause constant, intractable pain that radiates along the course of the nerve.

Gross appearance

Neurinomas are usually 1–4 cm in diameter and rarely exceed 8 cm. The principal exceptions to this rule are mediastinal and retroperitoneal neurinomas, which can expand into the body cavities and attain enormous proportions. In our experience, many of these cases are true fibromas and the diagnosis of neurinoma is arguable (Cervós-Navarro and Stoltenburg, 1975). The consistency of neurinomas is typically firm and rubbery, although they can be cheesy or crumbly. They are typically grey to white in colour, and the cut surface shows a whorled appearance with a variable amount of haemorrhage, cystic change or lipid deposition. depending upon the extent of degeneration within the tumour. The neural origin of a neurinoma is usually obvious in those lesions arising from peripheral nerves and nerve roots. When the nerve of origin is recognized, the tumour usually projects from one side and is adherent to the nerve. In large retroperitoneal and thoracic neurinomas the nerve of origin often cannot be found.

Microscopic appearances

Antoni (1920) described the two types of tissue that commonly occur in neurinomas; each type can be more or less sharply defined. The Antoni A tissue is characterized by compactly arranged spindle cells with long oval nuclei and indistinct cell membranes in H. and E.-stained sections; the cells

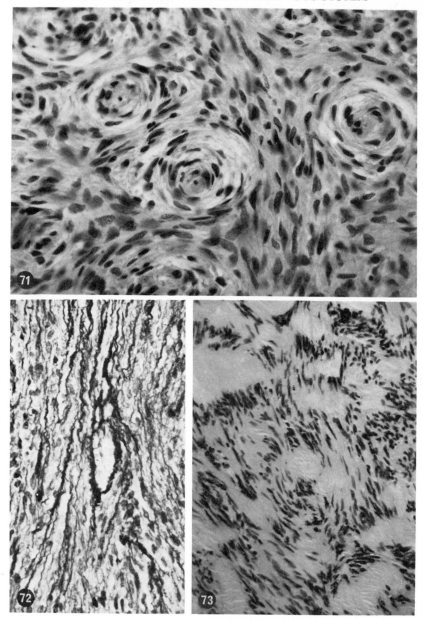

Fig. 71. Acoustic neurinoma in a 40 year old woman. Antoni type A tissue. Elongated spindle-shaped cells are arranged in interlacing fascicles and whorls. H. and E. stain; × 240

Fig. 72. Neurinoma (same case as Figure 71). The reticulin fibres in Antoni type A tissue run parallel to the surfaces of the tumour cells and exhibit a saw-tooth pattern. Reticulin stain; × 200

Fig. 73. Neurinoma of the sensory root at T 8 in a 34 year old man. Antoni type A tissue. The nuclei are arranged in palisades and separated by cytoplasmic processes. H. and E. stain; × 180

tend to be arranged in long sheets, interlacing fascicles and whorls (*Figure 71*). Occasionally, the nuclei are arranged in palisades that are separated by sheets of fibrillar cytoplasmic processes that are free of nuclei (*Figure 73*). While the palisades are by no means universally present in these tumours, they are quite distinctive and are better-defined than similar palisades that occur in other tumours. After silver carbonate impregnation, the neurinoma cells have slender elongated nuclei and two long polar processes arranged in parallel rows. Reticulin stains reveal fine undulating argyrophilic filaments in the Antoni A areas, some with a saw-tooth appearance running parallel to the margins of the tumour cells (*Figure 72*). Collagen is sparse except for fibrous bands that occasionally penetrate the tumour from the capsule.

The Antoni B tissue is loosely textured and free of fibrillar background (*Figure 74*). Individual cells are twisted, elongated or round in shape; they have distinct cytoplasmic margins and are widely separated by a matrix that stains poorly with H. and E. and is seldom positive for mucopolysaccharides with alcian blue (*Figure 75*).

Degenerative changes are present in both types of neurinoma tissue; they consist of focal aggregations of foam cells (*Figure 76*) containing sudanophilic lipid, and iron pigment in macrophages resulting from old haemorrhages. Well-marked vascular changes may occur, including dilatation of blood vessels, focal fibrinoid necrosis of the vessel walls, thrombi of varying ages and hyaline thickening (*Figure 77*).

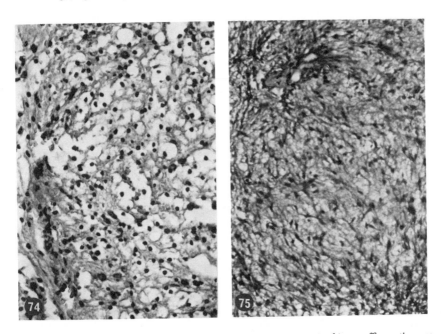

Fig. 74. Acoustic neurinoma, Antoni type B tissue. The clear spaces in this paraffin section are partly artefactual and cannot be demonstrated to the same degree in epoxy resin-embedded material. H. and E. stain; × 190

Fig. 75. Acoustic neurinoma. Mucoid material stained by cresyl-violet fills the microcystic spaces. Nissl stain; × 190

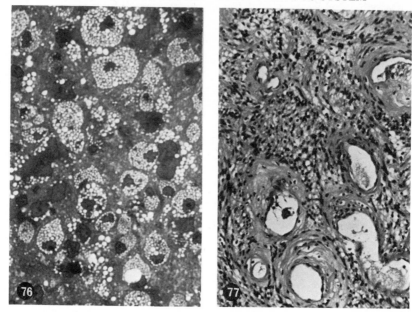

Fig. 76. *Acoustic neurinoma. Lipid-filled foam cells in an Antoni type A area. One micron epoxy resin section. Toluidine blue stain; × 500*

Fig. 77. *Neurinoma of the peroneal nerve. Antoni type B tissue with hyalinized blood vessel walls. The vessel at top right shows a hyalinized, organized thrombus occupying two-thirds of the lumen. H. and E. stain; × 120*

Electron microscopic appearances

The neurinoma cells in Antoni A areas have a tendency to form cytoplasmic processes by folding their plasma membranes (*Figure 78*). Although there is a certain amount of variation, as a rule every neurinoma shows this structural pattern in its cytoplasmic processes (Cervós-Navarro, Matakas and Lázaro, 1968). The processes lie close together and wrapped around each other. Some of the cytoplasmic processes do not exceed 100 nm in width and thus appear as a membranous system. The outer borders of such a membranous system are enveloped by continuous basement membrane.

The nuclei of the tumour cells in the solid fibrillary Antoni A areas are mainly elliptical and possess a finely granular nucleoplasm with dense areas mainly associated with the nuclear membrane (*Figure 79*). The nuclei usually have a smooth profile. As a rule the mitochondria are scarce and small; they possess few cristae and a dense matrix. There is considerable variation among these tumours in the amount of endoplasmic reticulum; most commonly it is sparse but in some tumour cells it is well developed.

Occasionally the space enclosed by the membranes of the endoplasmic reticulum is dilated and filled with electron-dense material. Free ribosomes are present in almost all tumour cells, even in those areas of cells which show little or no endoplasmic reticulum. In some cases the free ribosomes are distributed

160

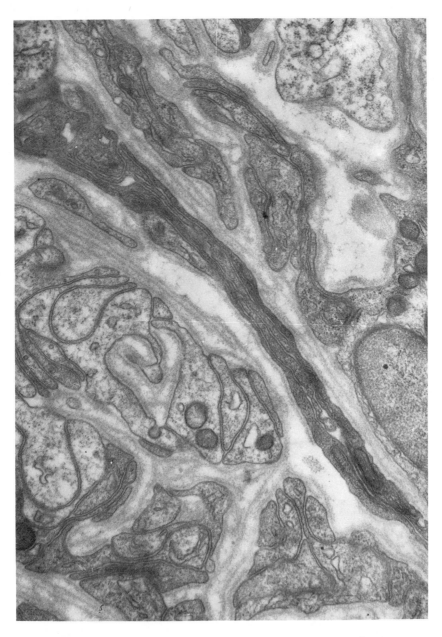

Fig. 78. Neurinoma (same case as Figure 71). Antoni type A tissue. Cytoplasmic processes formed by folding of the plasma membranes lie closely arranged and wrapped around each other. They are enclosed by basement membrane except where the adjacent plasma membranes are in close contact. Multilayered basement membranes are seen in the interstitial spaces. Electron micrograph × 30 000

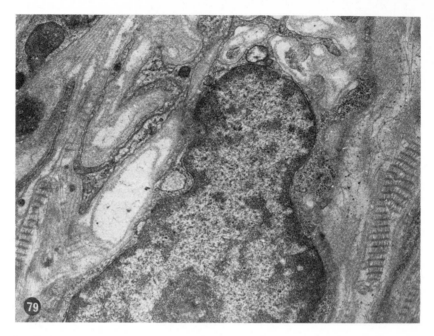

Fig. 79. Acoustic neurinoma. Transition from Antoni type A to Antoni type B tissue. The nucleus is surrounded by a narrow band of cytoplasm, and the expanded interstitial space contains microfibrils, filament bundles and multilayered basement membranes. Electron micrograph × 18 000

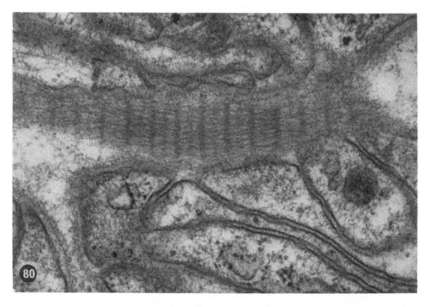

Fig. 80. Neurinoma (same case as Figure 71). High-power of periodic filament bundle. Two light bands and a central dense band are seen between the major dense bands. Electron micrograph × 45 000

162

throughout the entire cytoplasm, forming polysomes. Golgi-zones are regularly found in the perinuclear cytoplasm; the associated centrioles can be in the form of diplo- or sometimes also of triplosomes. Occasionally, ciliary stumps and rudimentary cilia are present. Filaments are seen to a varying degree in the cytoplasm of the neurinoma cells, and in glutaraldehyde-fixed material they may appear as microtubules. Cytosomes are seldom observed in typically Antoni A areas.

The extent of the interstitial space is very variable in different areas of Antoni A tissue in the same tumour; it can be so small that neighbouring cells appear to be separated by only a single basement membrane, but in the more extensive interstitial spaces there are multilayered basement membranes (*Figure 78*). Microfibrils and filament bundles are also seen in the interstitial spaces (*Figure 79*). The filament bundles were first described by Luse (1960) and are considered typical but not pathonomonic for neurinomas; they exhibit a spindle-shaped, or wide-banded profile and are generally round in cross-section. They can achieve a length of 7 µm and a width of up to 600 nm. In some tumours they are extremely uncommon and consist only of small bundles containing a few filaments. Single filaments have a diameter of about 10 nm, with a longitudinal periodicity of light and dark bands. The distance between two dark bands is about 140 nm; between these two bands two other light areas can be found, each about 50 nm wide and separated by a central medium-dense band (*Figure 80*). Most of the filament bundles showing this periodicity are found in areas rich in basement membrane material or near-collagen fibres. Some are enwrapped by cytoplasmic processes of the tumour cells (*Figure 81*).

Variations in the histological pattern of the tumour lead to the definition of Antoni type B tissue. The series of steps in the development of this tissue retain

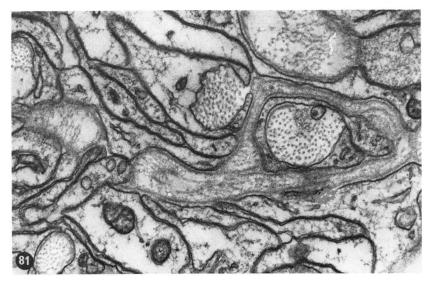

Fig. 81. Acoustic neuroma. Bundles of collagen fibres are enwrapped by cytoplasmic processes of the tumour cells with the formation of a 'mesocollagen'. Electron micrograph × 20 000

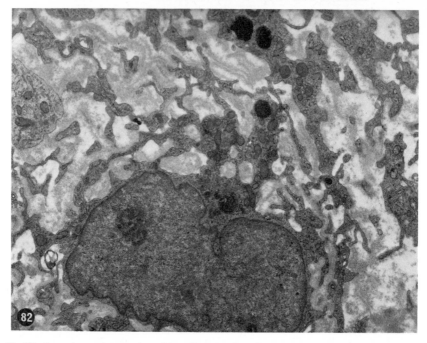

Fig. 82. Acoustic neurinoma. Antoni type B tissue. Cytoplasmic processes are slender and lack close contact with each other. The expanded interstitial spaces are filled with amorphous material and fragments of basement membrane. Electron micrograph × 12 000

the same structural principles as the rest of the tumour. In some cases the difference lies in the fact that the tumour cells move together at the expense of the interstitial space and display a reduction in their cytoplasmic processes. At the same time, the tumour cells become more rounded. In these areas single desmosomes occur sporadically and large numbers of cytosomes may be seen. In most cases, however, there is widening of the interstitial spaces, which are occupied by compact bundles of collagen fibres or (*Figure 82*) by amorphous material similar to basement membrane.

Comparing the light and electron microscope pictures of the Antoni B tissue, one finds that the light microscopically identifiable microcystic areas have no adequate ultrastructural equivalent (Matakas *et al.*, 1971). In 1 μm epoxy resin sections distension of the intercellular spaces is hardly ever as large as it seems in paraffin sections. The reticular structure of the neurinoma, therefore, appears to be mainly due to the tissue shrinkage that occurs with paraffin embedding. However, the fact that tissue shrinkage can have such a remarkable effect is probably explained by the relatively large size of the intercellular space. Above all, the cells in the Antoni B tissue can be distinguished from those in the fibrillary Antoni A areas by the fact that the cytoplasmic processes have much less contact with each other. Only rarely do the cell processes envelop each other in the Antoni B areas. Furthermore, the cells are rounded, and have only a few processes and a large perinuclear area; they are mostly widely separated and lie as narrow islands in the surrounding interstitial space.

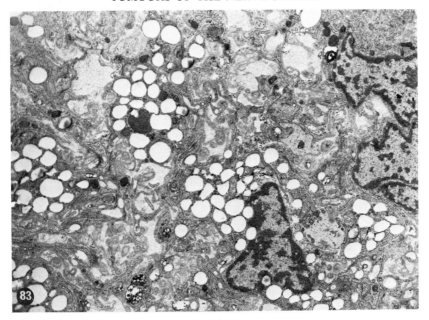

Fig. 83. Neurinoma (same case and area as Figure 75). In spite of the abundant lipid storage, the structural characteristics of the neurinoma cells are still recognizable. Electron micrograph × 5000

The cell nuclei in the Antoni B tissue sometimes show cytoplasmic invagination. Mitochondria are sparse and vary in size; the granular endoplasmic reticulum is not highly developed and is sometimes distended by electron-dense masses. The number of free ribosomes is usually low. Golgi zones are frequently seen, and occasional vesicles and saccules, often widely dilated, are also present. Cytoplasmic filaments occur in considerable numbers, and clumps of glycogen granules are seen in a few of the tumour cells. Cells containing lipid droplets are found in circumscribed areas in many tumours, in both Antoni A and Antoni B areas. In some tumours the lipid storage is so pronounced (*Figure 83*) that Müller (1965) suggested that it was part of an active metabolic process within the cells rather than the degenerative feature; the ultrastructural pattern of these cells is no different from that of the other neurinoma cells.

The large number of cytosomes which are found in the tumour cells of the Antoni B tissue is worthy of note (*Figure 84*). They are about 200–300 nm in diameter and at times considerably larger. Their profile is always almost round, and in contrast to the droplets of lipid material, they are bordered by a single outer membrane. At times, cytosomes contain light and dark circular inclusions. In a few tumours phagosomes are also present.

The amount of basement membrane in the areas of type B tissue is decreased. In the transition areas between Antoni A and B tissue a single basement membrane surrounds the tumour cell, but in the type B areas this often disappears. The intercellular space is then either filled by amorphous material or appears empty in electron micrographs. Basement membrane

165

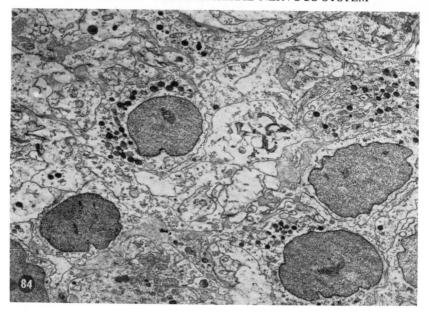

Fig. 84. Acoustic neurinoma. Antoni type B tissue. The tumour cells are rounded and close together; there is a reduction in the interstitial space. The cells contain large numbers of dense bodies (cytosomes) in the cytoplasm. Electron micrograph × 4000

material is more abundant in those areas which still retain a type A cellular structure but where the intercellular spaces are nevertheless expanded. Collagen fibrils are either single or in small bundles; sometimes they are arranged in a parallel fashion and display a pattern similar to that of the cross-banded filament bundles. The banding, however, has a periodicity of about 75 nm and the filament bundles with a periodicity of 140 nm seen in the type A areas are rarely found in type B tissue. Focal accumulations of microfibrils are distributed throughout the expanded intercellular space.

In addition to the typical cell forms in the spindle-shaped (type A) and the reticular (type B) areas, there is another kind of cell which is occasionally seen throughout the tumour. These cells have few processes and no basement membrane; the endoplasmic reticulum is highly developed and the cytoplasm is very pale, and they show no tendency to wrap around other cells. From these features they can clearly be classified as fibroblasts, but their origin from another type of endoneurial cell is also possible. These cells are not as common in neurinomas as they are in traumatic neuromas and neurofibromas.

Pathogenesis and differential diagnosis

The ultrastructure of neurinomas presents a number of features which suggest that these tumours arise from Schwann cells. The distribution and structure of the cell organelles are of less importance for the support of this hypothesis than is the fact that almost all tumour cells in type A tissue are totally surrounded by basement membrane; the cells in type B tissue are rather more variable in their basement membrane coating (Pineda, 1965; Wechsler and Hossmann, 1965; Cravioto, 1969). The hypothesis seemed less conclusive after Röhlich and Knoop (1961) showed that perineurial cells are also enveloped by basement membrane. Because of the presence of collagen in neurinomas, Raimondi and Beckmann (1967) concluded that these tumours are of fibroblastic origin; this supports the original contention of Penfield (1932), Tarlov (1940) and other authors. Harkin and Reed (1968), on the other hand, consider the perineurial cell to be a form of Schwann cell, and, consequently, adhere to the single term 'Schwannoma' for the common form of benign nerve sheath tumour of that name; they postulate that it may arise from either or both of these cell types. The equation of a Schwann cell with the perineurial cell has still to meet with general acceptance, particularly as most of the neurinomas arise in the roots of cranial and spinal nerves which have no coating of perineurium (McCabe and Low, 1969; Haller and Low, 1971).

Feigin (1971) has suggested that Schwann cells are specialized mesenchymal elements, but the evidence for this unitary mesenchymal concept is not conclusive, even though Murray and Stout (1942) showed that neurinoma cells *in vitro* are capable of producing collagen. Evidence has also been provided by Nathaniel and Pease (1963) that Schwann cells have the ability to polymerize collagen. As fibroblasts in neurinomas are rare or non-existent, it is difficult to consider these tumours as fibroblastomas purely on the basis of their collagen content.

Recent ultrastructural investigation of neurinomas has shown that the argyrophilic reticulin fibres do not represent a uniform substance within the tumour (Cervós-Navarro and Matakas, 1975). Reticulin fibres represent either basement membrane or the amorphous material frequently found in the interstitial spaces of neurinomas; microfibrils may also be part of the argyrophilic reticulin.

The conclusive proof for the origin of neurinoma cells from Schwann cells lies in the characteristic growth pattern displayed by the tumour cells where the processes enfold each other and tend to imitate the normal growth pattern of Schwann cells (Cervós-Navarro, 1960).

The relationship between type A and type B tissue in neurinomas has been discussed extensively since it became clear that they belonged to one tumour category. Light microscopical techniques, however, failed to elucidate the morphological connections between the two forms of tissue. Electron microscope findings, on the other hand, show quite clearly that the properties which distinguish type B tissue are modifications of a single tumour cell type; such modifications are mainly, but not all, of a degenerative nature. Degenerative changes such as hyalinization and fatty degeneration can also be found in areas of Antoni A tissue. Evidence for loss of normal Schwann cell function in the Antoni B tissue lies in the failure of the cells to form the stacked cell processes typical of Schwann cells. There is also a lack of collagen invagination, a process which is thought to reflect the ability of normal Schwann cells to ensheath axons. The sparse basement membrane formation in Antoni B areas with only partial covering of the cell surface again suggests cellular dedifferentiation (Matakas and Cervós-Navarro, 1969).

The distinction between neurinoma and neurofibroma is certainly the most common difficulty in the diagnosis of the two tumours; although many pathologists do not separate neurinoma and neurofibroma, such differentiation is possible and necessary; it will be outlined below (p. 175).

In neurinomas that involve the spinal cord and posterior cranial fossa it is important to know the exact location of the tumour, especially if a histological diagnosis is to be made on the basis of a frozen section. The histological pattern of gliomas of the central nervous system may closely resemble that of a neurinoma. In the gastrointestinal tract leiomyomas histologically resemble neurinomas, but leiomyomas are usually uniformly cellular and do not show the mixture of cellular areas and loose reticular tissue seen in neurinomas. Myofibrils may be demonstrated in the cytoplasm of smooth muscle cells with phosphotungstic acid haematoxylin stains.

Granular cell neurinomas

Synonyms: Granular cell myoblastoma; granular cell Schwannoma; granular cell tumour.

The origin of this tumour is unknown. While opinion remains divided, there is good evidence for the inclusion of granular cell 'myoblastoma' as a tumour in the Schwann cell family. Some recent reports favour a nerve sheath origin (Fisher and Wechsler, 1962; Rafel, 1962; Harkin and Reed, 1969), but other authors continue to favour a mesenchymatous origin (Moscovic and Azar, 1967). The tumours are most often solitary, but they can be multiple and are

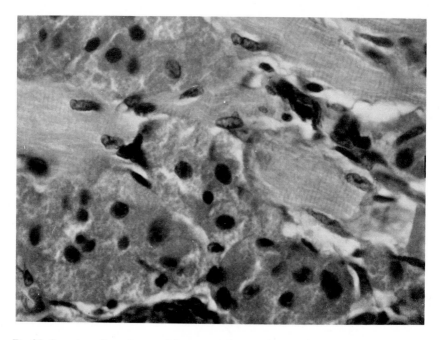

Fig. 85. Granular cell neurinoma of the tongue. The muscle fibres are separated by tumour cells which are plump and polygonal in shape; their cytoplasm contains many acidophilic granules.
× 560

usually benign. Some of the cases with multiple granular cell tumours in various organs reported as 'malignant granular cell myoblastoma' probably represent tumours of multifocal origin rather than metastases. Other lesions reported as malignant granular cell tumours are probably alveolar soft part sarcomas, rhabdomyosarcomas or melanomas. Approximately one-third of these tumours arise in the tongue, but they also occur very frequently in areas which characteristically possess no striated muscle (e.g. skin and breast).

The tumours are made up of large acidophilic polyhedral cells which exhibit a characteristic cytoplasmic granularity (*Figure 85*). The cells are arranged in compact interlacing fascicles. The granules in the tumour cells stain with periodic acid Schiff (PAS) stain and the basement membranes are prominent in tissue stained with silver impregnation methods for reticulin and with the PAS stain. At the deep margin of the tumour a fascicular arrangement is often prominent, and small peripheral nerves can be found in the tumour. Continuity between tumour cells and nerves is seen in both superficial and visceral lesions.

The cells have a consistent ultrastructural appearance (Sobel *et al.*, 1971). A basement membrane, similar to that of Schwann cells, can be found around some of the tumour cells. They have numerous closely packed cytoplasmic processes, a feature also seen in 'hypertrophic' Schwann cells. Cytoplasmic granules in granular cell tumours are unlike the 'granules' found in Schwann cells of nerves undergoing Wallerian degeneration.

NEUROFIBROMA

Synonyms: Nerve sheath tumours; neurinoma; Schwannoma: neuroblastomatosis; neuromatosis; plexiform neuroma; perineurial fibroma.

There are many questions concerning neurofibromas on which different authors disagree; it has therefore been difficult to evaluate the literature on these lesions.

The first question to ask is whether there is a real distinction between neurinoma and neurofibroma. Many authors deny such a difference and group both tumours under the same name (Zülch, 1955; Schmincke, 1956; Pineda, 1965; Cravioto, 1969). In a review of 264 cases Heard (1962) suggested grouping the lesions as follows: (1) neurilemmona (neurinoma) representing the encapsulated lesions; (2) neurofibroma, an unencapsulated neurinoma but of identical origin; (3) von Recklinghausen's disease, reserved as a term for cases demonstrating nodules, pigmented lesions, bony changes and a family history. Electron microscopy has clarified this issue and shown that both solitary neurofibromas and the lesions of von Recklinghausen's neurofibromatosis have well-defined structural differences from neurinomas (Luse, 1960; Waggener, 1966; Poirier, Escourolle and Castaigne, 1968).

The second question is whether solitary neurofibromas do occur, a point that Russell and Rubinstein (1963) doubted, or whether these tumours always associated with multiple neurofibromatosis. As Harkin and Reed (1968) pointed out, there is a mild forme fruste (incomplete or primitive form) of multiple neurofibromatosis, but this should not be overdiagnosed, particularly as the majority of patients with solitary neurofibromas of the skin have no other evidence of von Recklinghausen's neurofibromatosis. One further point is that single neurofibromas are indistinguishable from the individual tumours of von Recklinghausen's disease. As solitary tumours, neurofibromas are undoubtedly uncommon compared with neurinomas; therefore, when a diagnosis of neurofibroma has been made, the clinician is obliged to search for other manifestations of generalized neurofibromatosis.

The third question is whether neurofibromas can occur in the main sites of neurinoma formation, i.e. cranial and spinal nerve roots. Scharenberg (1971) and other authors make no distinction between solitary neurinomas and the tumours occurring in these sites in multiple neurofibromatosis. Gardner and Frazier (1930), Penfield (1932), Tarlov (1940) and others, however, found the characteristic histological pattern of neurofibromas in bilateral acoustic nerve tumours in patients with generalized neurofibromatosis. In our material we have a solitary neurofibroma arising in the posterior spinal root at C_3.

Incidence, location and clinical data

Because of the lack of specific identity of neurofibromas in the literature, no attempt will be made to characterize the incidence and clinical data of possible neurofibromas occurring at the same site as neurinomas. The age of onset for many of the lesions in cases of neurofibromatosis is variable; it ranges from new-born to old age, with two peaks of incidence at the age of 10–20 years and 50–70 years. The disease may not become fully developed until adult life, and some cases have shown an accentuation of the disease during pregnancy, which suggests an endocrine effect.

Neurofibromas themselves seldom cause pain or other symptoms, and the

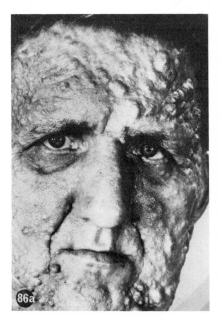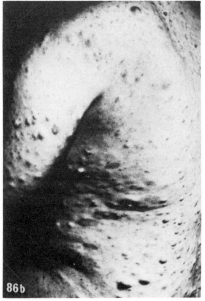

Fig. 86. Fifty-seven year old patient with von Recklinghausen's neurofibromatosis. Numerous cutaneous neurofibromas cover the entire skin of the face (a) and body (b)

tumour is often recognized simply because of its bulk. This is particularly so when the tumour arises in the neck, tongue or pharynx, where it may interfere with function. In the gastrointestinal tract neurofibromas often cause pain which simulates an ulcer, or they give rise to bleeding and diarrhoea. In cases of von Recklinghausens's neurofibromatosis the entire surface of the body may be covered with tumours (*Figure 86a,b*).

Cutaneous neurofibromas are sessile or pedunculated tumours; the former are to some extent mobile and moderately firm and rubbery. Neurofibromas may occur at any site along the peripheral nerves, but are more common in the deep major nerves, in retroperitoneal tissue and in the gastro-intestinal tract. In a survey of 168 cases of neurofibromatosis with impairment of gastrointestinal function, 51·7 per cent were localized in the small intestine, 21·4 per cent in the stomach, 11·3 per cent in the rectum, 8·3 per cent in the colon and 1·7 per cent in the appendix (Orcel, Luboinski and Natali, 1972). The thickened tortuous nerves are often described upon palpation as resembling a 'bag of worms'.

Gross appearance

Neurofibromas of the nerve trunks are fusiform, indistinctly encapsulated tumours inseparable from the nerve itself (*Figure 87*). The exact relationship of

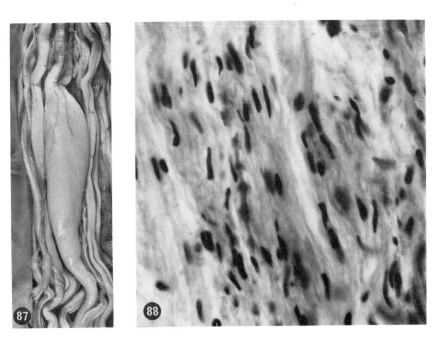

Fig. 87. *Fusiform neurofibroma of a spinal root in the cauda equina of a 62 year old woman. The tumour does not compress the nerve fascicle which remains within the blastomatous, thickened nerve*

Fig. 88. *Neurofibroma of the sciatic nerve showing a preserved myelinated fibre and the proliferation of plump spindle cells embedded in a fibrillary myxomatous background. H. and E. stain; × 370*

171

the tumour to the nerve is difficult to determine. If a nerve is seen entering a neurofibroma, it disappears into the substance of the tumour and is not stretched over the surface of the mass. The fascicular pattern remains and is often in a tangled form (plexiform neurofibroma).

Neurofibromas of the skin are well circumscribed but not encapsulated. If the tumours are encased in tissue that is otherwise normal, the limits are usually difficult to define, but in instances where the plexus of tortuous cords is embedded in a fibrous matrix the tumour may appear circumscribed.

The lesions are soft and elastic in comparison with the firm, rubbery consistency of neurinomas; the plexiform type are clearly distinguished by their knobbly, macaroni-like feel. Microscopic inspection of the cut surface reveals linear fascicles rather than the whorled appearance of neurinomas; neurofibromas exhibit little discoloration or degenerative features.

Microscopic appearances

The structure of a neurofibroma often resembles that of the nerve from which it originates. All the elements of the nerve are present, but arranged in a distorted and bizarre fashion (*Figure 88*). Nerve fibres, both myelinated and unmyelinated, are frequently found running through the substance of the neoplasm. The main tumour cells are fusiform, often twisted and usually compactly arranged in thin cords. Bipolar and multipolar cells with slender, long processes with occasional branches can be recognized in preparations stained with Del Rio Hortega's silver carbonate method and in 1 μm epoxy resin sections. Occasionally a neurofibroma has regions which resemble the Antoni type A tissue of a neurinoma. The differentiation between neurinoma and neurofibroma may be uncertain on the basis of light microscopy; however, there are no palisades, and pigmentation from old haemorrhages and foam-cell accumulations are far less conspicuous than in neurinomas. The prominent intercellular component of the neurofibroma is composed of numerous collagen fibres and of a well-organized matrix which usually stains with toluidine blue for mucopolysaccharides. The numerous collagen fibres in the matrix can be seen in reticulin-stained preparations where the silver-impregnated fibres are orientated in loose, somewhat irregular streaming patterns, or arranged in parallel thick bands. Such large amounts of collagen usually impart a more fibromatous appearance to these tumours than is seen in neurinomas (*Figure 88*). Also, in contrast to neurinomas, neurofibromas do not generally have markedly thickened arteries or contain cysts. Neurones from involved ganglia may be included in the neurofibromatous tissue without such a tumour being a neuroblastoma. In the gastro-intestinal tract, however, nerve cells from the plexuses of Auerbach and Meissner form part of the tumour; these lesions have been described as ganglioneuromatosis (Dahl, Waugh and Dahlin, 1957).

Electron microscopic appearances

With the electron microscope neurofibromas are seen to consist of a profusion of Schwann cells and nerve fibres surrounded, as a rule, by wide interstitial spaces (*Figure 89*). A large number of nerve fibres can be

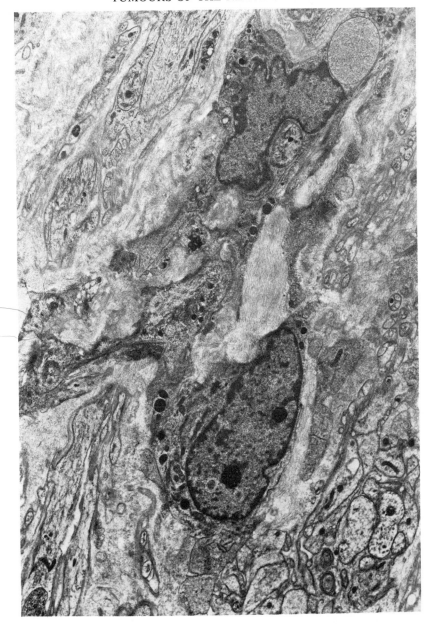

Fig. 89. Neurofibroma of the skin (same patient as Figure 86). Schwann cells and nerve fibres in a complex arrangment. The interstitial spaces contain tightly packed collagen fibres. Electron micrograph × 5500

identified throughout the tumour specimen, and at the periphery of the tumour the myelinated axons are often arranged in a similar pattern to that found in normal peripheral nerves. In the more central regions of the tumour myelinated fibres degenerate, whereas scattered non-myelinated axons may remain. The preserved axons are invaginated into the Schwann cells in a variety of ways; often the axons are only partly coated by a Schwann cell process or are in very loose contact with the Schwann cell (*Figure 90*).

The Schwann cells exhibit a wide variation in shape and size. Nuclei may be quite irregular in outline, and the chromatin is clumped along the nuclear membrane and in patches throughout the nucleoplasm. Relatively small amounts of cytoplasm surround the nucleus, but as a rule Schwann cells ensheathing myelinated axons have fairly large nuclei and abundant cytoplasm. Aggregates of microfibrils, a few mitochondria, Golgi apparatus, free ribosomes and granular endoplasmic reticulin profiles are all present in the cytoplasm. Not every Schwann cell is enclosed in a basement membrane; in some cases basement membrane ensheaths the cell on one side but not on the other. Cell processes with distinct basement membrane may also be found.

Elongated cells are scattered throughout the tumour (*Figures 91* and *92*); they are broad in the perinuclear region and have a few slender cytoplasmic processes which are highly irregular in shape and occasionally branched. Free ribosomes are the only organelles observed in the most distal regions of the processes. Bundles of fine filaments observed in the perinuclear region can be followed for variable distances into the proximal parts of the processes. The elongated cells do not possess a basement membrane, but since the basement membrane around Schwann cells in neurofibromas is not always rigidly applied to the surface, differentiation between the two cell types may be difficult.

Mast cells form a third cell type which is distributed diffusely throughout the

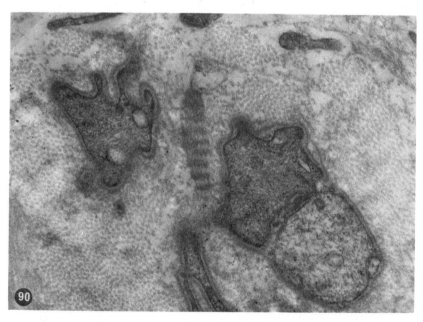

Fig. 90. Neurofibroma of the sciatic nerve. A non-myelinated axon runs beside a Schwann cell process but is not invaginated by it. Both axon and Schwann cell are surrounded by basement membrane. Tightly packed collagen fibres and a periodic microfibrillary bundle are seen in the interstitial space. Electron micrograph × 20 000

174

tumour (Isaacson, 1976). These cells are easily recognized by their electron-dense granules and fine cytoplasmic projections from their surface (*Figure 92*). Mast cells in neurofibromas have a similar appearance to mast cells in normal nerves and in the rest of the body (see Chapter 3).

The interstitial space varies in size and content among the different tumours and among the different areas of the same tumour. It contains electron-lucid homogeneous substances intermingled with denser amorphous material which is frequently drawn out into microfibrils and fibrillary bundles (*Figures 90 and 91*). Occasionally, fragments of basement membrane are observed detached from the cellular structures (*Figure 92*). The amount of collagen in a tumour is proportional to the size of the extracellular space; in some areas only a few scattered slender cell processes are observed embedded in dense bundles of collagen fibres.

Pathogenesis of neurofibromas

Despite the differences between neurinoma and neurofibroma, accumulated data on these tumours favour the concept that the Schwann cell is the main blastomatous component in both tumours. Most definite evidence for a close relationship between neurofibroma cells and Schwann cells is the observation that tumour cells are closely applied to axons in a similar pattern to that seen with normal Schwann cells and axons (Pineda, 1966). On the other hand, the

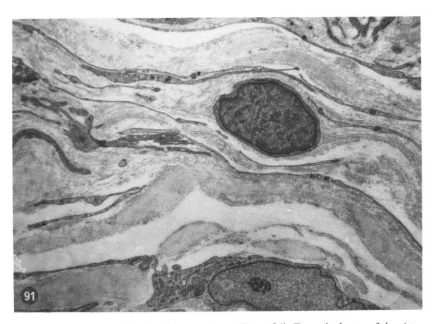

Fig. 91. Neurofibroma of the skin (same patient as Figure 86). Towards the top of the picture there is a Schwann cell with the nucleus surrounded by a thin rim of cytoplasm and ensheathed by a basement membrane. At the bottom there is a spindle cell with elongated cell processes devoid of basement membrane. The interstitial space is composed of electron-lucid homogeneous layers alternating with dense bundles of collagen fibres and slender cell processes. Electron micrograph × 5000

175

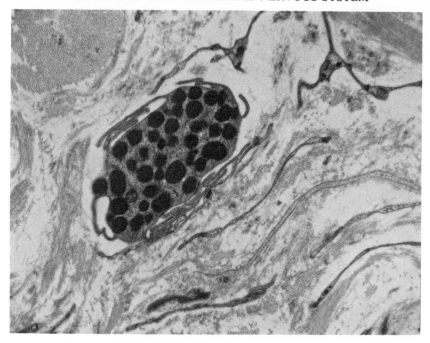

Fig. 92. Neurofibroma of the skin (same patient as Figure 86). Part of the extensive interstitial space containing a mast cell, fragments of basement membrane, microfibrils, collagen fibres and slender cell processes. Electron micrograph ×6000

tumour cells in neurofibromas have lost their capacity to accurately surround the axon and to form the characteristic infolding of their own processes. Furthermore, they may lack a basement membrane, and from this aspect they are rather similar to the tumour cells in the Antoni type B tissue of neurinomas. However, the latter cells have no relationship to axons, as these are absent from neurinomas except at the periphery. The fatty degeneration and lysosomal accumulation seen in Antoni type B tissue of neurinomas are uncommon in neurofibromas.

From light microscope observations it has been assumed that the axons found in neurofibromas are not neoplastic but trapped during growth of the tumour and by the proliferation of cells and increased production of matrix (Harkin and Reed, 1969). There is some evidence from electron microscopy, however, that axons growing in neurofibromas are an active blastomatous component of the tumour, and may not, in fact, just be trapped by the proliferation of Schwann cells and collagenous matrix.

As the constituent elements of neurofibromas are the same as those of a normal nerve, including nerve fibres, some authors consider neurofibromas to be dysplastic rather than blastomatous in nature (Rubinstein, 1963; Zülch, 1963; Poirier, Escourolle and Castagne, 1968). Because of the large amount of collagen in neurofibromas, a fibroblastic origin, or at least a fibroblastic component for neurofibromas, has been favoured by some authors (von Recklinghausen, 1881; Penfield, 1932; Adair and McLean, 1937; Tarlov,

1940). However, as reported above, there is now strong evidence that Schwann cells can produce collagen; thus, the principal reason for favouring the fibroblast as the cell of origin is no longer convincing. It seems probable, therefore, that the few fibroblasts and mast cells in neurofibromas are not, in fact, tumour cells; this view has been stated by many authors who have studied neurofibromas with the light microscope (Del Rio Hortega, 1943; Polak, 1950).

The bipolar and multipolar cells with elongated processes correspond to some of the cells described by light microscopy as lemnocytes (Del Rio Hortega, 1942). In an ultrastructural study Pineda (1966) stated that the presence of basement membranes around many of the cells suggests their probable derivation from Schwann cells. Poirier et al. (1968), on the other hand, identify some of these cells as fibroblasts. It is significant that similar processes can be found in traumatic neuromas (*Figure 63*), and it is possible that in many cases these cells have a perineurial or endoneurial origin. From light microscope studies it is thought that, in the early stages, the neoplastic process is confined to the perineurium except in those tumours which arise from the small terminal nerve branches. The lack of basement membrane, on the other hand, suggests an endoneurial (fibroblast) origin. Despite the uncertain origin of the tumour cells, the number of fibroblasts in neurofibromas has been largely overestimated in the literature.

In neurofibromatosis there may be an associated overgrowth of the soft tissue surrounding the hypertrophied nerve trunks; in severe forms the skin and soft tissue in the involved area may hang in thick, loose folds (elephantiasis nervosa). In cases where the neurofibromas involve the gastro-intestinal tract all the constituents of the intestinal wall are involved in the hyperplastic process. These observations favour the hypothesis that the genetic defect in neurofibromatosis is related to the increase in nerve growth factor recently demonstrated by Schenkein et al. (1974). The effect of the genetic defect, however, is not limited to nerve, and when enlargement of a finger or the appendix is occasionally present in patients with neurofibromatosis (localized hypertrophy), the constituent nerves show few, if any, changes.

Multiple mucosal neuromas

Synonyms: True neurinoma; myelinic mucous neuroma; Rankenneuroma.

Up to the present time some 20 cases have been reported in the literature where there has been a combination of multiple neurogenic tumours affecting mucous membranes. They have occurred chiefly on the conjunctiva, eyelids, lips and tongue (*Figure 92*), and involvement of nasal and laryngeal mucosa has also been described (Thies, 1964). Tumours may appear at all these sites or in any combination of sites; a mixture of mucosal and cutaneous tumours has also been described (Thies, 1964; Schnitzler et al., 1973). The age incidence of reported cases ranges from 8 to 42 years (mean age, 25 years). Tumours in the eyelid and tongue are described as small and hard; if the lips are involved, one or both lips may show diffuse hypertrophy. About half of the reported cases were associated with pheochromocytomas which were occasionaly bilateral (van Epps, Hyndman and Greene, 1940; Braley, 1954) and in some cases with thyroid carcinoma (Williams and Pollack, 1966).

This syndrome complex is obviously closely allied to von Recklinghausen's disease, particularly in the association of neural tumours with pheochromocytoma. In addition, there is the likelihood of an overlap with von Recklinghausen's disease in a case reported by Rappaport (1953). However, none of the patients is reported as having any relatives with the stigmata of von Recklinghausen's disease.

Histological examination shows that the tumours are composed almost entirely of nerve fibres with only a minimal fibrous component (*Figure 94*). The nerve fibres are arranged in bundles surrounded by thickened perineurium, and the bundles are haphazardly arranged, running in many different directions throughout the tumour. The histological pattern resembles that of a traumatic neuroma, but there is little collagen formation. Ganglion cells have been described in only one case (Braley, 1954). Electron microscopic studies have been reported in two cases (Schnitzler *et al.*, 1973; Cervós-Navarro and Thies, 1975), but there are no essential differences between the ultrastructural pattern of these tumours and that of neurofibromas in other sites. Myelinated fibres are present and non-myelinated axons are most conspicuous (*Figure 95*). There is a more exact correlation between axon and Schwann cells than is usually present in neurofibromas, but there is also proliferation of Schwann cells, which may be divorced from the nerve fibres and exhibit autonomous growth. The basement membrane is incomplete around these cells, and bundles of nerve fibres and Schwann cells are partially surrounded by endoneurial (*Figure 95*)

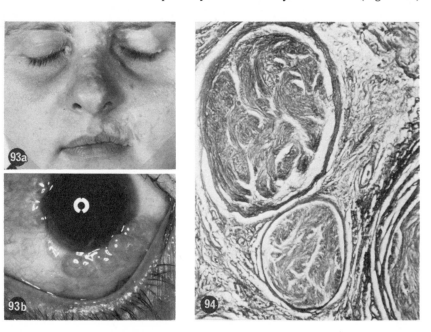

Fig. 93. Multiple mucosal and cutaneous neurinomas in a 25 year old woman. (a) Tumour nodules in the eyelids and on the skin of the nose and lips. (b) Multiple conjunctival neurinomas

Fig. 94. Same case as Figure 93, a lesion from the lip showing hypertrophy of the nerves cut in cross-sections. Bielschowsky stain; × 100

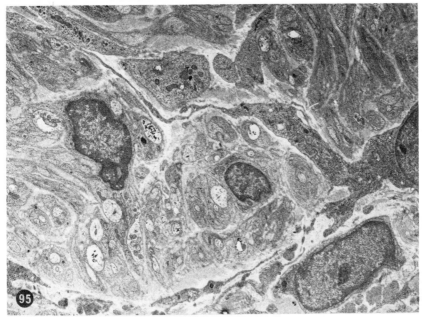

Fig. 95. Same lesion as Figure 94. There is proliferation of non-myelinated axons and Schwann cells. The latter surround the nerve fibres, but also show autonomous proliferation. Perineurial and/or endoneurial cells are also hypertrophic. The interstitial space is reduced. Electron micrograph × 5000

and perineurial cells. The interstitial spaces are usually small, but if enlarged, they contain bundles of thick, closely packed collagen fibres.

BENIGN TUMOURS OF THE NERVE SHEATH—SUMMARY

Despite the fact that neurinomas and neurofibromas are frequently not distinguished from each other in the literature, differential diagnosis between the two tumours should be simple on both electron and light microscopic examination. As the neurinoma grows, it compresses the nerve but does not incorporate the nerve fibres; it is locally confined and distinctly encapsulated. Neurofibromas, on the other hand, are not well demarcated, and they expand within the nerve and incorporate nerve fibres which participate in the blastomatous growth. In addition, there are certain features by which neurinomas are recognized, namely the characteristic palisading of nuclei and the presence of Antoni type A and type B tissue; these features are not present in neurofibromas. Ultrastructurally, the differentiation between the two tumours is even more clearly defined; this has been set out diagramatically in *Figure 96*.

MALIGNANT TUMOURS OF THE NERVE SHEATH

Synonyms: Malignant Schwannoma; malignant neurilemmoma; neuro-fibrosarcoma; neurogenic sarcoma; neurogenous fibrosarcoma; fibro-

179

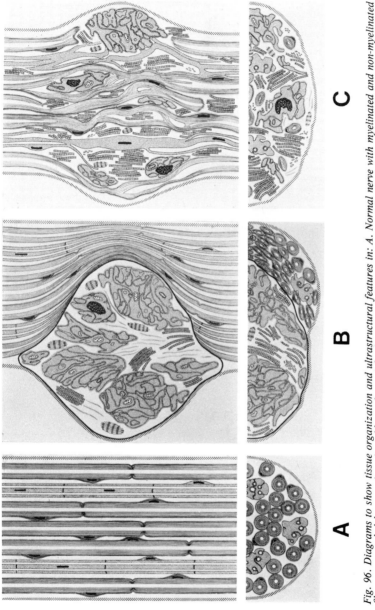

A

B

C

Fig. 96. Diagrams to show tissue organization and ultrastructural features in: A. Normal nerve with myelinated and non-myelinated fibres surrounded by a perineurium (the endoneurial compartment is not represented here). Schwann cells surround the axons; in myelinated fibres the cytoplasm of the Schwann cell can only be seen in the perinuclear region, whereas the Schwann cytoplasm is more prominent in those cells associated with non-myelinated fibres. In a cross-section at the lower part of the diagram, the mesaxons associated with the non-myelinated axons can be seen. The Schwann cells are coated by basement membrane. B. A neurinoma compressing the adjacent nerve fibres as it increases in size. The tumour is encapsulated and the main cellular components are neoplastic Schwann cells showing extensive enfolding of the plasma membranes. Large amounts of basement membrane are present in the interstitial spaces, together with periodic microfibrillary bundles and sparse collagen fibres. C. A neurofibroma expands within the nerve and is not encapsulated. The nerve fibres are not displaced to the periphery of the tumour mass but entwined within it. Only some of the blastomatous elements are derived from Schwann cells. The axons are involved in the disordered growth. The elongated processes of the Schwann cells are represented in the diagram but not those of possible endoneurial or perineurial origin.

180

myxosarcoma of nerve; fibrosarcoma myxomatodes; sarcoma of peripheral nerve; secondary malignant neuroma.

The group of tumours that has been reported as primarily malignant nerve sheath neoplasms is a remarkable and histologically varied one; consequently, the terminology for malignant tumours of nerve sheath origin is even more confusing than that for the benign tumours. Since the criteria for the differentiation between neurinomas and neurofibromas has been firmly stated above, it seems appropriate to propose the following classification for malignant tumours of the nerve sheath along similar lines.

Group (a): malignant neurinoma (malignant Schwannoma)
Group (b): malignant neurofibroma
Group (c): nerve sheath fibrosarcoma

Thus the tumours from Group (a) would originate from Schwann cells alone; those in Group (b) from Schwann cells, nerve fibres and perineurium or endoneurial elements; and those from Group (c) solely from fibroblasts of endoneurial or perineurial origin. However, the specificity of the microscopic pattern is not necessarily conclusive evidence for distinguishing malignant nerve sheath tumours of Schwann cell origin from fibrosarcomas or other mesenchymal sarcomas.

Because of their rarity and the lack of precise terminology, the available data on any of these tumours do not amount to a significant, established body of knowledge. The cases that have been studied ultrastructurally do not cover the above-mentioned histological varieties; a generally acceptable classification may be possible once further observations have been made. Until we have a better understanding of these tumours, we can only try to evaluate the available data in the literature and in our own material.

(a) Malignant neurinoma (malignant Schwannoma)

Despite the frequent diagnosis of malignant neurinoma (Schwannoma) in the past, and the inclusion of this tumour in the UICC classification, the histological characteristics of a neurinoma have not, as yet, been demonstrated in any malignant tumour. The most common histological feature in the various cases described as malignant nerve sheath tumours is the complete lack of any pattern that suggests an origin from a benign, solitary, encapsulated neurinoma. The characteristic palisading of nuclei and the presence of Antoni type A and Antoni type B tissues by which neurinomas are recognized are not present in the malignant tumours. Finally, the weight of evidence suggests that malignant neurinomas arise in peripheral nerves as single entities and their association with pre-existing benign lesions is coincidental. Benign neurinomas, however, are frequently misdiagnosed as malignant.

Russell and Rubinstein (1959) concluded that when a well-defined malignant spindle-cell tumour arises in the course of a nerve at a site favoured by benign neurinomas, there is reasonable argument for accepting it as a malignant tumour of Schwann cells. However, in contradistinction to benign neurinomas, cases reported as malignant neurinomas involve predominantly the deep nerves and have tended to favour the median and sciatic nerves;

malignant tumours rarely occur on the roots of spinal or cranial nerves. Malignant nerve sheath tumours can occur sporadically, without the manifestation of neurofibromatosis (D'Agostino, Soule and Miller, 1963), but their histological features of malignancy are more indefinite.

Often, when the term 'malignant neurinoma' or 'Schwannoma' has been applied in the literature, the differences between neurinoma and neurofibroma have been disregarded. However, now that these differences can be clearly defined, the majority of tumours diagnosed as malignant neurinomas should probably be classified as malignant neurofibromas. The well-defined ultrastructural characteristics of neurinomas have not been demonstrated in any malignant tumour. One of the rare cases of malignant transformation in a neurinoma that seems probable was reported by Carstens and Schrodt (1967) in a 93-year-old woman. Unfortunately, the pieces of tissue obtained for electron microscopic examination contained only benign tumour. As light microscopy of the malignant area showed a few pseudorosettes, the authors pointed out the possibility of a neuroblastomatous transformation.

(b) Malignant neurofibroma

Malignant tumours of peripheral nerves are well recorded in von Recklinghausen's disease. The incidence of malignancy in neural tumours in neurofibromatosis is variously estimated from 5 per cent (Preston, Walsh and Clarke, 1952) to 16 per cent (Stout, 1949). Reported series are probably not quite reliable with respect to such statistics, since patients with the mild forme fruste of neurofibromatosis are rather common and rarely receive medical attention.

Isolated malignant nerve tumours have been reported in all major areas, including the brachial plexus, neck, face, mediastinum, coeliac plexus, retroperitoneal tissue, pericardium and all major nerve trunks. Cutaneous nerves are often involved.

There is no characteristic symptomatology of this tumour and no symptom can be considered diagnostic. The chief reason why the patient usually comes for advise is the presence of a tumour mass. In those patients with von Recklinghausen's disease the recent, more rapid growth of a small mass, which may have been present without symptoms for a long time, causes the patient to seek aid because of fear that the growth has become cancerous. On the other hand, the size of the mass may start to cause pain or inconvenience. The tumour may have shown an increase in rate of growth or may have recurred rapidly after excision of a plexiform neurofibroma. Although it has been claimed that malignant transformation in multiple neurofibromatosis follows surgical procedures, there is little evidence to support this hypothesis.

Gross appearance

The gross features are essentially those of a neurofibroma of deep nerves. While most tumours arise in nerves, many demonstrate the same general appearance without a definite macroscopic relationship to nerves. Strict observance of the nature and degree of involvement of the nerve is indeed necessary, since extraneural soft tissue sarcomas may completely surround the nerve, may infiltrate the epinerium, and on rare occasions may actually invade the nerve longitudinally for short distances. Malignant neurofibromas present either as a fusiform enlargement of the nerve or as a single, lobulated, circumscribed mass. The growth may remain encapsulated or confined within the nerve sheath expanding it or forming a round or fusiform mass whose shape is determined by the denseness of the surrounding tissue into which the nerve tumour is expanding. In some cases the tumour may attain a large size without revealing any microscopic evidence of infiltration of surrounding tissues, whereas in other cases the tumour appears encapsulated to the naked eye, but the capsule is in reality a pseudocapsule. At the points at which this 'capsule' adheres to muscle, fascia, bone or vessels, the tissue can usually be shown histologically to contain viable tumour cells (Nieta and Pack, 1951).

Microscopic appearances

The structure of a malignant neurofibroma resembles that of a benign neurofibroma but with circumscribed, poorly differentiated areas. The nerve fibres within the tumour are mainly non-myelinated and the cellularity is higher than in benign tumours. In some areas the cells are plumper, tend to be pleomorphic and form a looser pattern with microcystic changes. In areas which retain some of the characteristics of a neurofibroma there are clusters of cells forming an epithelioid pattern with prominent mitotic activity. Blood vessel walls are hypertrophic and there is proliferation of cells in the perineurium. The less well-differentiated areas show mitotic activity and a paucity of background fibrillar substance (*Figure 97*). There may be a marked cellular infiltrate, suggesting an intense inflammatory response, which may lead to misdiagnosis. Rarely, metaplasia occurs, especially the formation of cartilage or bone. Reports of cases where a histologically questionable 'malignant neurofibroma' has metastasized may reflect the incomplete sampling of the specimens. One such tumour studied contained large areas which were best classified as a cellular neurofibroma and only small zones of obviously malignant neoplasm were present. It is usually possible to find areas of a pre-existing plexiform neurofibroma, and in some areas of the tumour, a gradual transition to malignant neurofibroma can be demonstrated. Palisading of cells around areas of necrosis, similar to that seen in primary tumours of the central nervous system, is a feature that has been emphasized as characteristic of malignant peripheral nerve tumours (Harkin and Reed, 1969).

Electron microscopic appearances

There are few reports of malignant nerve sheath tumours in neuro-fibromatosis (Gonzalez *et al.*, 1964; Matakas *et al.*, 1971). In these reports it has been stated that the ultrastructure of the neoplastic cells differs from that of the neurofibroma and that they should be considered as fibrosarcomas. In a single case studied by us the neoplasm was composed of Schwann cells, some of which contained axons, but, in addition, there were non-myelinated axons that were not always associated with Schwann cells. As a rule, Schwann cells as well as

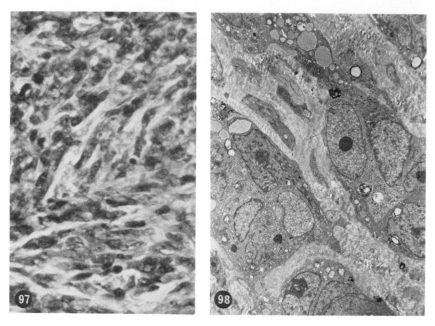

Fig. 97. Malignant neurofibroma. A poorly differentiated area with high cellularity and a paucity of fibrillar background. H. and E. stain; × 350

Fig. 98. Malignant neurofibroma (same case and area as Figure 97). Clusters of Schwann cells are growing in an epithelioid arrangement without the inclusion of axons. Electron micrograph × 2800

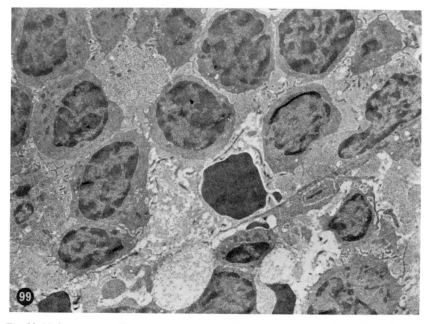

Fig. 99. Malignant neurofibroma (same case as Figure 97). Another field of an undifferentiated area with a cellular infiltrate suggesting an inflammatory response. Ultrastructurally the cells resemble monocytes. Electron micrograph × 3700

184

axons were enveloped by basement membrane. Schwann cells not associated with axons may proliferate in clusters (*Figure 98*), producing a pattern that has been described as the ultrastructural equivalent of the cellular Schwannoma (Paquin and Mandelenakis, 1973). The cells found in the collagenous matrix of the tumour, in the vicinity of the cell clusters or Schwann cell axon complexes, gradually lose the characteristics of Schwann cells and can no longer be differentiated from fibroblasts.

There is considerable proliferation of blood vessels and of their cellular components. Large arterial vessels show hypertrophy of the muscle cells in the media, but development of elastic fibres is very poor in the subintimal region and non-existent in the media; connections between the loosely arranged smooth muscle cells are not observed and a regular adventitial layer is missing. Other vessels show a dilated lumen and a thin endothelial wall similar to that seen in sinusoids. Some areas of the vessel walls show proliferation of muscle cells which do not form an organized medial layer but spread out into the surrounding intercellular collagenous matrix. As they spread further from the blood vessel wall, the smooth muscle cells tend to lose the characteristic dark patches on the surface membrane and to develop more endoplasmic reticulum; also, in the course of this process, they lose their basement membranes. Similar cells develop from the pericytes around small blood vessels and thus do not go through the smooth muscle cell stage. In both cases the cells lying in the collagenous matrix show the characteristics of fibroblasts, and many have lipid droplets within the cytoplasm.

For the most part, the interstitial space in these tumours is filled with densely packed collagen fibres. The tumour cells within the collagenous matrix appear, at first, to have been trapped during the laying down of the collagen

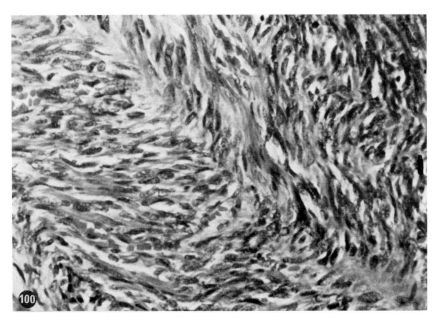

Fig. 100. Fibrosarcoma of a nerve sheath. Spindle cells are arranged in interlacing bundles producing a herring-bone pattern. H. and E. stain; × 320

185

bundles, but it is more probable that they are in fact invading the connective tissue. Ultrastructural studies of the cellular infiltrates, which by light microscopy suggest an inflammatory response, show that the cells are lymphocytes and monocytes (*Figure 100*). The cells have little or no endoplasmic reticulum, and the plasma membranes show numerous pseudopodia and folds.

(c) Fibrosarcoma of the nerve sheath

Nerve sheath fibrosarcomas are the most common type of malignant neoplasm found in association with neurofibromatosis. The majority of malignant tumours of the nerve sheath described in the literature should really be included in this group despite the original term ascribed to them. Although the tumour cells are thought to be fibroblasts, it is not known whether the lesion may be in part, or totally, derived from perineurial or endoneurial cells. Confusion arises because, on the one hand, the Schwann cell is capable of producing collagen, and on the other hand, the microscopic appearances of malignant neurofibromas is very similar to that of fibrosarcoma. The specificity of the microscopic pattern is not necessarily conclusive evidence for distinguishing malignant nerve sheath tumours from fibrosarcomas or other mesenchymal sarcomas.

Circumscribed masses attached to a nerve are not necessarily always a tumour with primary origin in that nerve. On the other hand, malignant tumours in patients with multiple neurofibromatosis may arise in relation to nerve trunks or within soft tissue independent of the nerves. In most instances the soft tissue involvement occurs in close association with a matted mass of proliferating mesenchymal tissue and plexiform neurofibroma. When a malignant tumour develops in such a mass of tissue, it is difficult to determine the locus of origin, as the tumour has infiltrated across the structural barriers in the area. Sarcomas may arise in the thigh in association with elephantiasis neuromatosa and may present as circumscribed tumours in diffuse neurofibromatosis.

D'Agostino, Soule and Miller (1963) found that only 6 of 21 malignant tumours in neurofibromatosis arose within a nerve trunk; they were situated in the sciatic nerve, brachial plexus, femoral nerve and the posterior tibial nerve. The remaining 15 tumours showed no gross or microscopic evidence to prove that any of them arose within the nerve trunk. In several reports it has been stressed that tumours in this category are highly malignant; they recur locally after excision and may metastasize. However, by dating the patient's survival from the reputed recognition of the tumour rather than from the day of treatment, Hitchens and Platt (1972) found that fibrosarcomas of various origins, including that of the nerve, have a low-grade malignancy.

Gross appearance

The gross appearance is not distinctive; it resembles many other sarcomas. The surface of the tumour mass may have a bluish tinge because of the numerous small blood vessels coursing over it. Some tumours are circumscribed, grey and firm, with obvious whorling and interlacing fascicles on their cut surface, whereas others are soft and contain cystic and haemorrhagic areas of degeneration; not infrequently, these two patterns are combined in the same tumour. In cases where a tumour has recurred at the same site following surgery, it may consist of a lobulated, eccentric mass both within and outside the nerve; in the majority of cases, however, the tumour is well-circumscribed and confined within the involved nerve. Infiltration of the tumour both proximally and distally along the nerve and its branches may occur, and in other cases some of the tumour may infiltrate into the surrounding soft tissue.

Microscopic appearances

Histological sections reveal unequivocal evidence of malignancy within the tumour with invasion of the epineurium. The tumour itself is composed of small, spindle- and oval-shaped cells tightly packed and arranged in interlacing bundles interspersed with a reticulin network. Sheaths of tumour cells produce whorls and a herringbone pattern (*Figure 98*). In many areas the cells are loosely arranged and are separated by a mucinous matrix. Stains for reticulin often reveal different patterns within the same tumour; silver-stained fibrils may form coarse parallel strands which separate the rows of spindle-shaped cells (named by Stout 'straight wire reticulin fibres'), whereas in adjacent parts of the tumour the cells are entwined by delicate reticulin fibres. D'Agostino, Soule and Miller (1963) have observed the same two forms of reticulin pattern on many occasions in malignant spindle-cell tumours that show no evidence of having arisen within a nerve. Hence, the reticulin stain has been of no practical assistance in differentiating fibrosarcoma of the nerve sheath from fibrosarcoma of other origin.

A similar morphological pattern in tumours in the intestinal tract has caused confusion between benign and malignant tumours of smooth muscle and malignant nerve sheath tumours. The demonstration of myofibrils in the cytoplasm of the tumour cells has resulted in the recognition, by most pathologists, that the majority of spindle-cell tumours arising in the gastro-intestinal tract are of smooth muscle origin.

Electron microscopic appearances

At low magnifications numerous cells are visible sectioned in longitudinal, transverse and oblique planes. The longitudinally sectioned cells exhibit an irregular outline and are spindle-shaped, with long, thin polar projections. For the most part, the long cellular projections are arranged parallel to one another and in some fields these cells constitute the major cellular component. Occasionally, a single fine, irregular projection arises from the surface of the cell. More frequently, the cellular outline is irregular and undulating. Transversely sectioned cells exhibit an irregular circular contour. In some areas intercellular junctions of the zonulae adherentes type can be seen; more commonly, however, neighbouring cells and their processes are separated from one another by clefts of varying width filled with a cloudy, finely granular or delicately fibrillar substance. Sometimes this material forms an extracellular

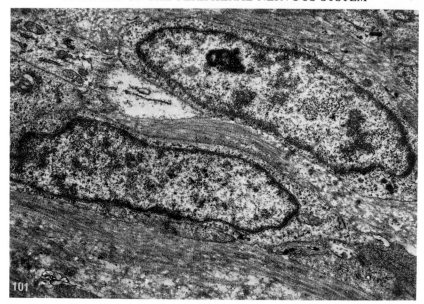

Fig. 101. Fibrosarcoma of the nerve sheath. Spindle-shaped cells in longitudinal section; the large nuclei have prominent nucleoli. Elongated processes are arranged parallel to each other and the interstitial space contains densely packed collagen bundles. Electron micrograph × 14 000

layer of basement membrane-like material applied to the cell surface, but no distinctly formed basement membrane surrounding the entire cell is present. The nucleus is centrally placed in the cell and in longitudinal section shows irregular, wavy indentations. Occasionally, single deep invaginations of cytoplasm into the nucleus are also observed. Large nucleoli are seen and the nuclear chromatin is evenly distributed, with a narrow rim of marginal condensation. The main characteristic features in the cytoplasm are the abundance of fine filaments and the well-developed rough surface endoplasmic reticulum. Broad bundles of filaments arranged in a parallel fashion occupy a considerable area of some cells, and appear to displace the other cytoplasmic organelles. Mitochondria are few in number and the Golgi apparatus is usually well-developed; ribosomes and polysomes are loosely scattered throughout the cytoplasm. The perinuclear regions and peripheral parts of the cell are usually more richly endowed with cellular organelles, especially rough surface endoplasmic reticulum. Pinocytotic vesicles are associated with the cytoplasmic membrane in some cells.

The interstitial spaces vary among different tumours and in different areas of the same tumour. There may be only granular and finely fibrillar proteins present with almost no collagen; however, usually most of the extracellular space is occupied by dense bundles of collagen fibres (*Figure 101*).

C. TUMOURS OF NERVE CELL ORIGIN

In the peripheral nervous system tumours of nerve cell origin occur predominantly in the region of the sympathetic trunk; this predilection is probably due to the embryological origins of the tumour cells. Sympathogonias are the stem cells not only of sympathoblasts and sympathetic ganglion cells but also of the chromaffin (pheochromic) cells found in the adrenal medulla and in coccygeal and carotid glands. Thus, two types of tumour occur in the sympathetic system which correspond to the dichotomy in the development of sympathogonias: (1) sympathetic tumours in the strict sense, arising from neuronal cell lines; (2) pheochromocytomas, arising from chromaffin (pheochromic) cells.

Pick and Bielschowsky (1911) divided the sympathetic neuronal tumours into three types, reflecting three developmental phases of normal ganglion cells in the sympathetic nervous system. The sympathicogonioma and sympathicoblastoma represent immature tumours; the ganglioneuroma represents the mature type. The terminology used in the literature shows no uniformity; most frequently the immature types of tumour, i.e. the sympathicogonioma and the sympathicoblastoma, are called neuroblastomas.

The tumour may contain cells at different stages of development, and this is used as a criterion for grading malignancy of the tumour. Beckwith and Martin (1968) graded these tumours from I to IV; Grade I corresponds to the most undifferentiated, whereas Grade IV is the most differentiated tumour. This may be justified if a distinction is to be made between ganglioneuroma, on the one hand, and ganglioneuroblastoma (malignant ganglioneuroma), on the other. In a review of the cases in the literature, however, we could find no substantial differences between the descriptions of ganglioneuroma and ganglioneuroblastomas; therefore, unlike the UICC classification, we do not distinguish between these two tumours. In our experience, on the other hand, the distinction between sympathicogonioma and sympathicoblastoma is justified on histological grounds. Although a mixed cell population can be found in these tumours, classification according to the major cell type present is usually not difficult. However, as the distinction between sympathicogoniomas and sympathicoblastomas has been practically abandoned in the last two decades, these tumours will be described together under the heading of neuroblastoma.

Recent biochemical studies have demonstrated that sympathetic tumours in the strict sense are able to synthesize and secrete catecholamines—a characteristic which is well known in pheochromocytomas. The amounts of catecholamines stored in individual tumours, however, have been reported as being quite variable. Variability has also been noted in the excretion rate of urinary catecholamines and their metabolites in patients with these tumours (Robinson, 1966; Goldstein, 1966). Until now, no definite correlation has been found between tumour catecholamine content, urinary catecholamine excretion and tumour type. The available data, however, were obtained in studies where no distinction between sympathicogoniomas and sympathicoblastomas had been carried out, and all the immature nerve cell tumours were grouped as neuroblastomas. It may be expected that a more careful histological classification of these tumours would allow a better clinicopathological correlation.

Nerve cell tumours are extremely rare in the ganglia of cranial and spinal nerves. Reports by early authors of ganglioneuroma of dorsal root ganglia in neurofibromatosis are not convincing and are more properly interpreted as the entrapment of ganglion nerve cells in neurofibromas. Neuroblastomas and ganglioneuromas of the Gasserian ganglion seem to be the only ones which are well substantiated (Döring, 1955).

NEUROBLASTOMA

Synonyms: Sympatheticogonioma; sympatheticoblastoma; immature sympathetic cell tumour; malignant ganglioneuroma.

Neuroblastomas occur primarily in the sympathetic nervous system. In more than half the cases they arise from the adrenal glands or the neighbouring coeliac, mesenteric or other abdominal ganglia. The remainder of the tumours develop in the sympathetic chains and rarely from the peripheral ganglia in the viscera or perivascular plexuses. In about one-half of the reported cases the patients have been less than 2 years old, and nearly three-quarters of the cases are less than 4 years old (Willis, 1948). The mature type of tumour (sympatheticoblastoma) occurs later in childhood or in young adults. Neuroblastomas of both mature and immature type, however, occur at any age, and if a congenital origin of neuroblastoma is postulated, it is necessary to assume that the tumours lie dormant for prolonged periods or have vastly different growth rates; neither of these assumptions seems probable. In a large series of 76 neuroblastomas Barrons (1957) found that the adrenal was the site of neuroblastoma in 51 per cent of the patients under the age of 3 years; it was the primary site in 35 per cent of patients in the 3–14 year age group; and the primary site in only 13 per cent of adult patients.

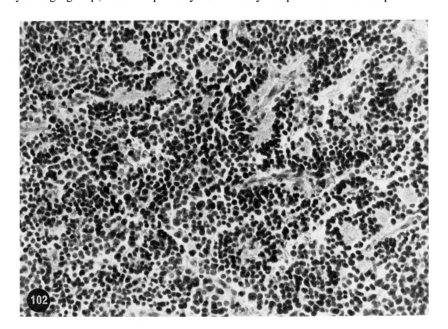

Fig. 102. An undifferentiated retroperitoneal neuroblastoma (sympathicogonioma) in a 7 month old child. Closely packed neoplastic cells are seen with rosette formation. H. and E. stain; × 240

Gross appearance

The size of the tumours varies from less than 1 × 1 cm to a massive growth which occupies most of the abdominal cavity. They are pale grey and dark red and may be sharply demarcated in some regions but fade into the adjacent tissue in other areas; necrosis, haemorrhage and cyst formation are all common features. Small tumours may be encapsulated, whereas the larger tumours have either an incomplete capsule or no capsule at all. Neuroblastomas are highly malignant and tend to metastasize. The base of the skull and the orbital bones are very often the sites of bone metastases; in very rare instances the primary lesion may occur in the orbit where it originates from the ciliary ganglia (Skydsgard, 1944).

Microscopic appearances

Typical histological appearances are seen in the majority of tumours grouped together as sympatheticogoniomas; the neoplastic cells are relatively uniform, with scanty cytoplasm and round-to-oval nuclei with diffuse granular chromatin. The cell margins are usually difficult to define, and mitotic figures are present. There is close packing of the neoplastic cells, with minimal interstitial elements. The cells tend to be arranged in a circle around a central

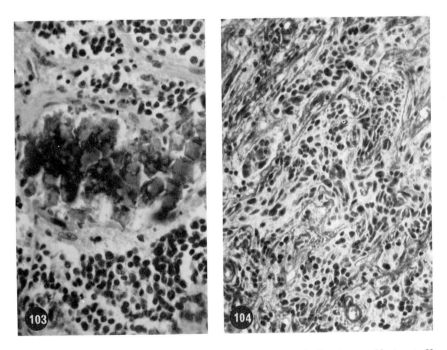

Fig. 103. Same case as Figure 102. Calcification is a common finding in neuroblastomas. H. and E. stain; × 280

Fig. 104. A well-differentiated neuroblastoma (sympathicoblastoma) of the mediastinum in a 2 year old child. The tumour cells have abundant cytoplasm and are separated by numerous nerve fibres. H. and E. stain; × 280

mesh of tangled cell processes (*Figure 102*)—a pattern that has been called both rosette and pseudorosette. The rosettes range from 40 to 50 μm in diameter; they are present in about 50 per cent of cases (Stowens, 1957) and are often emphasized as a diagnostic feature, but areas of fibrillary cell processes within the tumour are at least as distinctive and are more common than rosettes (Harkin and Reed, 1968). These fibrillar areas resemble fibrin and are often misinterpreted as such. Many cells have small pyknotic nuclei and a moderate amount of nuclear debris. In large tumours there may be extensive areas of necrosis; small necrotic areas and scattered foci of calcification (*Figure 103*) are commonly found. In the more differentiated tumours (sympatheticoblastomas) the cells have more cytoplasm (*Figure 104*); the short processes of the unipolar and bipolar tumour cells can be demonstrated by silver impregnation techniques.

Electron microscopic appearances

Three major ultrastructural patterns (types A, B and C) can be distinguished in neuroblastomas. In the undifferentiated tumours (sympatheticogonioma), as in the case of Tazawa, Soga and Ito (1971), only type A areas are found. The more mature tumours (sympatheticoblastoma) contain all three types of ultrastructural pattern.

In the type A pattern (*Figure 105*) the tumour cells are loosely attached to one another and the cell interfaces are relatively smooth, with fine, undulating

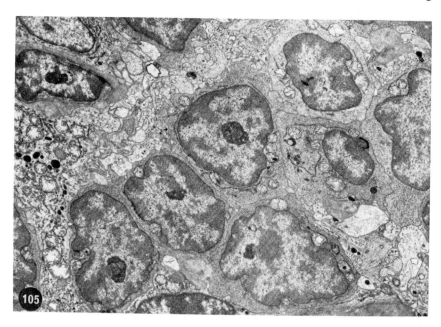

Fig. 105. Type A area of the same neuroblastoma as Figure 102. Polyhedral tumour cells have a thin rim of cytoplasm around the nucleus. There are few cytoplasmic processes within the cluster of cells but they are more numerous at the periphery (top left of picture), where the tissue merges with a Type B area. Electron micrograph × 7000

surfaces devoid of interdigitations; a few desmosomes, however, are apparent. The nuclei are round, eliptical or polygonal; occasionally, they have cytoplasmic invaginations. When well-fixed, the nucleoplasm is finely granular, with a few condensed zones, mostly located at the periphery; the nucleoli are prominent and large. The perinuclear cytoplasm usually forms a narrow ring around the nucleus and contains only a few organelles such as free ribosomes and scattered mitochondria. Golgi cisterns and rough-surfaced endoplasmic reticulum are poorly developed, but occasionally there are aggregates of cytoplasmic fibrils. Pseudopodia are rare, but when observed, they contain few organelles and are only present in a limited area of the free cell surface.

In the type B areas (*Figure 105*) tumour cells are separated by numerous islands of cytoplasm which are actually tangential sections of cytoplasmic processes. Occasionally, several neoplastic cells are arranged in a rosette-like pattern in the centre of which there are cytoplasmic processes of varying size. The nuclei of the tumour cells are smaller than in type A areas and are more irregular, with occasional cytoplasmic invaginations and deep clefts of the nuclear membrane; the chromatin patterns and nucleolar structures, however, do not differ from type A tissues. There is a well-developed rough-surfaced endoplasmic reticulum in the cytoplasm, together with numerous free ribosomes and large numbers of mitochondria; hyperplastic forms of mitochondria can be found scattered throughout the cells in this area. Golgi zones are better developed in the type B cells. In contrast to the cells of type A areas, where few cell processes are present, abundant cytoplasmic processes are observed in the type B tissue cut in both longitudinal section and cross-

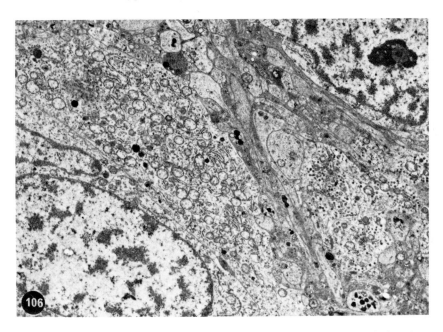

Fig. 106. Type C area of the same neuroblastoma as Figure 105. Tumour cells have large amounts of cytoplasm with well-developed endoplasmic reticulum and large numbers of mitochondria. Dense-cored vesicles are seen in the cell at the top left of the picture. Electron micrograph ×15 000

section. These processes are clearly seen to be extending from the cell body in instances where they are sectioned longitudinally. Some of the processes are pale-staining, while others resemble axons and contain small, dense-cored vesicles; cell organelles are also present in the cytoplasmic processes and microtubules run parallel to their long axes.

The cells of type C areas (*Figure 106*) have polymorphic nuclei with prominent nucleoli. There is more cytoplasm associated with these cells than in the type A and B areas. The endoplasmic reticulum is well-developed and there are large numbers of mitochondria; not infrequently, the cytoplasm contains numerous, round, dense-cored vesicles, ranging from 100 to 400 nm in diameter. These granules are homogeneous, osmiophilic and membrane-bound. Larger granules are also present, but they are irregular in shape and size and occasionally more than 1 µm in diameter; they vary in their internal structure, some being finely granular, whereas others contain myelin figures.

Numerous nerve fibre processes are seen in sections of type C tissue, and in some areas these nerve fibres are arranged in broad bundles (*Figure 107*). The nerve fibres also frequently contain small, dense-cored granules. In addition, some large dense-cored vesicles are seen; they are approximately 500 nm in diameter. Large numbers of membrane-bound dense bodies are observed in some processes, and, occasionally, many microtubules (30–35 nm in diameter) and neurofilaments are seen arranged parallel to the long axis of the nerve fibres.

Synapse-like structures in neuroblastomas have been described by Luse (1964), Misugi, Misugi and Newton (1968) and Yokoyama (1971). Other authors have been unable to confirm these structures in neuroblastomas

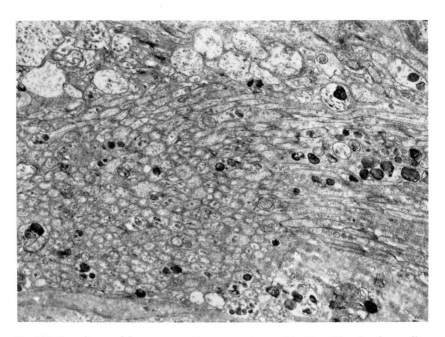

Fig. 107. *Type C area of the same neuroblastoma as Figure 106. A broad bundle of nerve fibres contains large dense-cored vesicles and dense bodies. Electron micrograph × 15 000*

(Yanagisawa, 1970). Despite the large number of cell processes in some of our tumours, no indisputable synaptic structures have been observed in our cases.

Cells with laminae formed from plasma membranes have been described by Yokoyama *et al.* (1971). As similar structures have been described in oligodendrogliomas and malignant blue naevi, Yokoyama *et al.* (1971) have suggested that these peculiar cells may originate from Schwann cells. However, other authors who have studied the ultrastructure of neuroblastomas have concluded that typical Schwann cells are not present.

The tumour cells and cytoplasmic processes in neuroblastomas lack a basement membrane even where their cell surfaces border a perivascular space. Amorphous homogeneous material containing scanty collagen fibres and large numbers of microfibrils fill the intercellular spaces; microfibrillary bundles with a characteristic periodic striation are also seen.

Pathogenesis and differential diagnosis

Early in foetal life neuroblasts migrate from the neural crest and advance along the segmental visceral rami of the anterior spinal roots to the intramural plexuses of the viscera. Bielschowsky (1932) stated that the length of this route favours faulty cell development, resulting in immature cells potentially capable of proliferation. This could explain why nerve cell tumours in the peripheral nervous system, especially in the sympathetic nervous system, are much more common than nerve cell tumours in the central nervous system (Christensen, 1971). As neuroblastomas are neoplasms of embryonic tissue, it is logical that the incidence of tumours should be highest during the time that the formative tissues are present in the body. It is well known that the amount of embryonic neuroblastic tissue diminishes from the postnatal period until puberty (Beckwith and Perrin, 1963).

Since Cushing and Wolbach (1927) reported the transformation of a sympatheticoblastoma into a ganglioneuroma, the spontaneous regression of sympathetic nerve cell tumours as well as their differentiation has been extensively discussed. However, although the possibility of maturation of a 'neuroblastoma' into a 'ganglioneuroma' is one of the most debated and most intriguing features of the tumour, the actual number of cases in which this transformation has been demonstrated is small (Altermann and Schueller, 1970). On the other hand, in a follow-up review based on the histology of 66 cases of neuroblastoma, Greenfield and Shelley (1965) found 30 cases with clear evidence of maturation. Systematic studies have shown that, among all the malignant tumours, neuroblastomas have the highest rate of cure, differentiation and change in biological activity (Everson and Cole, 1966; Bill, 1968; Koop, 1968). Maturation within these tumours has been ascribed to changes in concentration of nerve growth factor in the serum (Varon, 1968) or to immunological processes (Coriell, 1968).

Neuroblastomas are often mistaken for lymphosarcomas; also, the obsolete term 'round cell sarcoma' has been and is still used for these tumours. An important characteristic in the differential diagnosis is the distribution of reticulo-endothelial cells (Polak, 1966); in the sympatheticogoniomas and sympatheticoblastomas these cells are scattered throughout the tumour, whereas in lymphosarcomas they are always grouped in nests.

Because of the presence of rosette-like patterns in Wilm's tumour, difficulties may arise in its differentiation from neuroblastomas. The frequent calcification in neuroblastomas is an important characteristic for differentiation, as this feature is always lacking in Wilm's tumours. Another source of confusion is Ewing's sarcoma. In fact, many cases described as Ewing's sarcoma may actually have been metastases from neuroblastomas; rosettes, however, never occur in Ewing's sarcoma.

Ganglioneuroma

Synonyms: Gangliocytoma; ganglioglioma; ganglioneuroblastoma.

Ganglioneuromas usually originate from ganglion cells of the sympathetic nervous system, although it is also probable that such tumours arise from sympathetic nerves as well as other peripheral nerves. They occur mainly in adults over 20 years of age, and in a series of 109 tumours Stowens (1957) found 39 patients older than 50 years. Cases of multiple ganglioneuromas have also been described and are thought to represent an unusual variant of von Recklinghausen's disease; this view is supported by the presence of café au lait spots, skin involvement and familial incidence in some patients.

The tumours are usually slow-growing and occur most commonly in the posterior mediastinum, retroperitoneal tissues, adrenal glands and sympathetic ganglia. Ganglioneuromas may occur as solitary lesions or, as mentioned above, they may be multiple; they vary in diameter from a few millimetres to several centimetres. Macroscopically, the tumours are white, firm and encapsulated, with a pearly-grey cut surface. As a rule, the tumours are benign and do not metastasize, but a few ganglioneuromas show local infiltration. Metastases from the encapsulated tumours and from the more apparent malignant representatives of this group of tumours may occur; they are found especially in the liver and in the base of the skull. If a tumour shows rapid growth but has a histological pattern of ganglioneuroma on biopsy, it should be suspected that the specimen is not representative of the whole tumour and that more primitive, malignant elements are also present.

Microscopic appearances

The mature ganglion cell is the hallmark of this tumour. Such cells occur in varying numbers and may be scattered singly throughout the tumour or arranged in clumps. The cells show some evidence of degeneration, and they are often surrounded by a capsule of satellite cells. The ganglion cells have moderately abundant eosinophilic cytoplasm and large vesicular nuclei. Multinucleate cells are commonly found in these tumours, especially in ganglioneuromas that have matured from neuroblastomas; each nucleus in these cells has a well-defined nucleolus. The degenerative changes in the ganglion cells are mainly pyknosis, cytoplasmic eosinophilia and particularly marked cytoplasmic ballooning; the latter cells may be three to four times the normal size and often contain clusters of finely granular lipofuscin in their cytoplasm. In some instances there is evidence of calcification of individual cells or groups of ganglion cells. There is an abundant, dense stroma which may contain stainable neurofibrils as well as collagen fibres, but the stromal pattern may vary considerably, and arrangements reminiscent of neurofibromas may be seen. Prominent lymphoid aggregates can occur in ganglioneuromas, either forming islands of cells or distributed as bands of small lymphocytes throughout the tumour; sometimes the lymphoid aggregates are grouped around small blood vessels.

Electron microscopic appearances

The tumour cells have large nuclei with prominent nucleoli measuring up to 2 μm in diameter. There is abundant cytoplasm which contains a complex arrangement of various organelles and inclusions. Mitochondria are present in large numbers and are occasionally irregularly shaped. Extremely large mitochondria measuring 1 μm in diameter are sometimes seen; they have cristae which are extremely short and well-defined (Gonzalez-Angulo, Reyes and Navarrete, 1965). Granular endoplasmic reticulum and smooth endoplasmic reticulum are frequently observed. Free ribosomes are scattered throughout the cytoplasm, occasionally forming a polysome arrangement. A well-developed Golgi complex is found in the perinuclear region.

Numerous granules of different shapes and sizes are present in the cytoplasm (Misugi *et al.*, 1968). The smaller granules are round, uniform in size and shape, limited by a membrane and filled with homogeneous osmiophilic material; they are about 100 nm in diameter and resemble catecholamine granules. These smaller granules are distributed throughout the perinuclear region and are frequently associated with the Golgi complex. The larger granules are generally ovoid but show considerable variation in shape and size, with diameter ranging from 250 nm to several hundred nanometres; they are also membrane-bound and contain homogeneous osmiophilic material. The small and large granules are frequently intermingled, and in some areas, the small granules are encircled by the large granules and appear to be incorporated into them; the granules frequently conglomerate to form still larger masses. Multivesicular bodies up to 300 nm in diameter are also seen in the cytoplasm of the tumour cells.

Much of the space between the tumour cell bodies is filled with bundles of cell processes of varying length. Some of the processes are surrounded by Schwann cells but others lack a Schwann sheath. Between the axons, there are abundant collagen fibres and cytoplasmic expansions of normal and atypical Schwann cells. One Schwann cell usually ensheaths several axons. Fine filaments and microtubules are seen in the axons, together with varying numbers of small and large granules similar to those seen in the perinuclear regions. In some areas, the neurites are expanded and contain accumulations of dense-cored granules about 100 nm in diameter and small, clear vesicles measuring 50–120 nm in diameter. Occasionally, there is an increase in the density of the plasma membrane at the point where expanded neurites make contact with a cell body or with other neurites. Typical synapses, however, have not been encountered in many of the tumours described (Yokoyama *et al.*, 1973).

Myelinated nerve bundles are occasionally present in some of the tumours;

such myelinated axons also contain neurofilaments, neurotubules, mitochondria, and dense-cored vesicles and granules. All the ganglion cells are in close contact with satellite cells and surrounded by them (Yokoyama *et al.*, 1973). In some areas, the cytoplasmic processes of the satellite cells are as thin as 100 nm or less, but the external surface of the cell is always covered by a basement membrane. Occasionally, basement membrane material is identifiable between the satellite cell and ganglion cell (Gonzale-Angulo, Reyes and Navarrete Reyna, 1965). The basement membranes around the nerve bundles have the same thickness as those surrounding ganglion cells. Varying quantities of collagen are interspersed among the ganglion cells and their bundles; fibrocytes are occasionally seen.

Pathogenesis and differential diagnosis

There has been considerable discussion in the literature about the origin of ganglioneuromas. Many authors have concluded that ganglioneuromas and maturing neuroblastomas are derived from mature ganglion cells which either maintain their maturity or dedifferentiate. They base their conclusions upon the morphology, clinical behaviour, age incidence and the sites of origin of the tumours within the sympathetic nervous system (Stowens, 1957). Greenfield and Shelley (1965), on the other hand, pointed out that ganglioneuromas consist of a rather orderly arrangement of ganglion cells and nerve fibres with covering Schwann cells, and it is difficult to believe that such a complex arrangement in large tumours could result from the division of mature ganglion cells. Furthermore, no tumour classified as a maturing neuroblastoma has shown any evidence that it arose by malignant transformation within a pre-existing ganglioneuroma. These points, therefore, favour the idea expressed by Willis (1959, 1960) that all ganglioneuromas, at some time in their histogenesis, have been neuroblastomas but that, as they have matured, they have lost their malignant potential.

Giant cell astrocytomas in the brain have not infrequently been misdiagnosed as ganglioneuromas. The differential diagnosis in the peripheral nervous system, however, is usually fairly easy, but if autochthonous nerve cells are trapped within a neurofibroma, the tumour may be mistaken for a ganglioneuroma (Bolande and Towler, 1970).

Pheochromocytoma

Synonyms: Chromaffin tumour; chromaffinoblastoma; chromaffinoma; paraganglioma; medullary adenoma of the adrenal; pheochromoblastoma.

A pheochromocytoma is a neoplasm of the adrenal gland which typically secretes adrenalin, noradrenalin or both. The tumour is usually found in the adrenal medulla and is bilateral in more than 10 per cent of cases. Interadrenal sympathetic ganglia are also fairly frequent sites for this tumour, and the thoracic sympathetic ganglia are occasionally involved.

Several syndromes are associated with pheochromocytomas; they include von Recklinghausen's neurofibromatosis, intracranial haemangiomas and multiple mucocutaneous neurinomas (Davis, Hull and Vardell, 1950; Chapman, Kemp and Taliaferro, 1959). Symptoms are present in only about 80 per cent of cases; they include paroxysmal or sustained hypertension, headache following exercise, paraesthesiae of the hands and feet, palpitations, dyspnoea, nausea, vomiting, epigastric pain, hyperglycaemia, tachycardia and blanching. The symptoms often occur in periodic attacks associated with elevation of plasma catecholamine levels. These attacks may last for minutes or hours and terminate with flushing of the blanched areas and sweating. The urinary catecholamines in patients with pheochromocytomas may reach levels of 10–100 times normal; paradoxically, the high values are observed between the paroxysmal attacks of hypertension.

Gross appearances

Pheochromocytomas vary in size from small microscopic lesions found incidentally to masses weighing over 2 kg; the average tumour, however, weighs 100 g and is 5–6 cm in diameter. The tumours are circumscribed, rounded, grey or red in colour and surrounded by a stretched adrenal cortex. Haemorrhages, cystic areas, calcification and central dense fibrous scars are commonly seen within the tumour.

Microscopic appearances

The tumour cells are most often round or polygonal in shape, chromaffin-positive and arranged in loose aggregates within a delicate connective tissue stroma. They are abundantly supplied with capillaries and the venules in an arrangement similar to that seen in the normal adrenal medulla. The round or oval nuclei contain fine, loosely meshed chromatin and minute nucleoli. Scattered swollen, misshapen nuclei are seen which contain coarse, irregular chromatin and huge nucleoli; this is considered to be a degenerative feature rather than an indication of malignant transformation (Mulligan, 1971). The cytoplasm of the tumour cells is granular and tends to be basophilic with formaldehyde fixation and polychromatophilic or acidophilic with chromate fixation. Areas of necrosis and cytstic change within the tumour may be observed. The periadrenal adipose tissue in cases of pheochromocytoma typically has an excess of brown fat (Melicow, 1957).

Electron microscopic appearances

The tumour cells are rounded or polyhedral and arranged in a compact fashion, usually separated from each other by a gap of only 20 nm. There may be some pleomorphism, and the numerous cell processes pass between the cells and interdigitate with processes of neighbouring cells (*Figure 108*). The nuclei are large, ovoid, with a smooth profile; binucleate and multinucleate cells are frequently seen. Although the nucleoplasm is mostly clear, there are some dense areas subjacent to the nuclear membrane.

For the most part, mitochondria are round and their cristae are sparse;

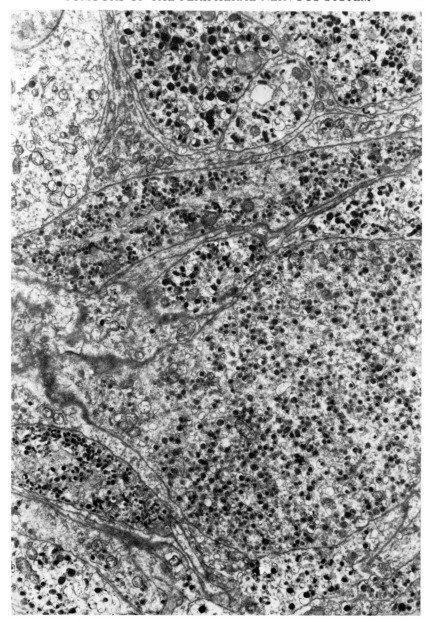

Fig. 108. Pheochromocytoma. The tumour cells and their interdigitating processes contain osmiophilic cytoplasmic granules of varying size and stage of development distributed irregularly throughout the different cells. Electron micrograph × 7000

occasional cells have large numbers of mitochondria. Much of the endoplasmic reticulum is agranular and is found mainly in the lightly stained cells, which are also rich in mitochondria; the granular endoplasmic reticulum has a more

200

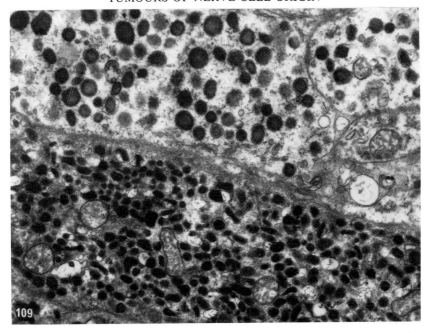

Fig. 109. Pheochromocytoma. Various cell types can be differentiated by the size of their granules. This is an unusual finding in pheochromocytomas but common in the normal adrenal medulla. Electron micrograph × 17 000

irregular distribution. Golgi complexes showing saccular dilatations are widely spaced throughout the cytoplasm of the cells that contain few granules; the granules in these cells are found within the Golgi zones. Very few Golgi complexes are seen in the cells that are rich in osmiophilic granules. Centrioles and diplosomes are often situated near the Golgi zones, and glycogen granules are scattered throughout the majority of the cells and occasionally form focal accumulations. Osmiophilic granules are seen in most cells; they are 100–300 nm in diameter and are circular or slightly elongated in shape (*Figure 108*). The granules vary in density; some cells only have the lighter-staining granules. Large circular osmiophilic granules with diameters of 500 nm or more are found occasionally. The distribution of the various types of granules in the tumour cells is, on the whole, irregular, so that individual cells contain granules of various shapes, size and density (Cervós-Navarro, Bayer and Käser, 1973). In only one of our six cases were various cell types distinguishable by the difference in size (150–400 nm), shape (round or elongated), number and density of their granules (*Figure 109*). In some pheochromocytomas we have found cells containing characteristic neuronal elements.

Small desmosomal intercellular junctions have been observed between the plasma membranes of tumour cells. The intercellular clefts are often distended and contain amorphous dense material which is the ultrastructural equivalent of the reticulin demonstrated by light microscopy (Cervós-Navarro and Matakas, 1975).

The capillaries in the tumour tissue are fenestrated and have pinocytotic vesicles in the endothelial cells; a broad basement membrane separates the chromaffin cells from the capillary endothelium.

D. TUMOURS OF NON-NERVOUS ORIGIN

Vascular malformations and vascular tumours of other organs are occasionally associated with von Recklinghausen's complex. Many Schwannomas and neurofibromas have a prominent vascular supply and the potentiality for angioblastic proliferation in such tumours has been noted (Barber, 1962; Krücke, 1974). Isolated tumours have seldom been described. Losli (1952) reviews seven cases of cavernous haemangiomas of nerves, two of his own and five in the literature. Barber (1962) and Krücke (1974) have described further cases. Haemangioendotheliomas involving peripheral nerves have been described by Naffziger and Brown (1933) and Stout (1949, 1953).

Direct extension of tumours into the perineurial spaces is usually taken as histological evidence of malignancy. Such extension of tumour cells along the nerve sheath or in the neural lymphatics is commonly seen with certain tumours (*Figure 110*), especially carcinoma of the prostate, leukaemias, lymphomas and even sarcomas. Secondary involvement of nerves by sarcomas arising in soft tissue in neurofibromatosis has been stressed as a major difficulty in the differential diagnosis of fibrosarcoma of the nerve sheath. Taylor and Norris (1967) have also described direct extension along

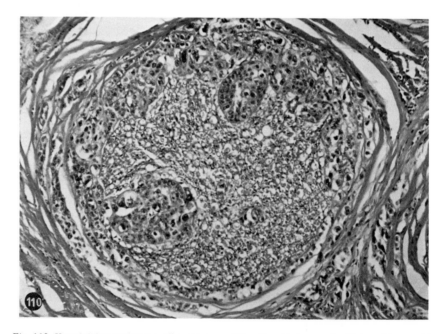

Fig. 110. Keratinizing squamous cell carcinoma of the ethmoid sinus and orbit in a 61 year old man. A nerve fascicle is involved but there is little compression of the neural structures. H. and E. stain; × 100

perineurial spaces in a benign process such as sclerosing adenosis of the breast. Hodgkin's lymphogranulomatosis not infrequently involves the vertebrae and spreads into the spinal roots (Birkel, 1971). Extension along major nerves is rather less common and has been reviewed in some detail by Willis (1952) in connection with the general relationship of nerves and malignancies.

Haematogenous metastases in peripheral nerves are extremely rare, but metastatic spread via the cerebrospinal fluid with attachment and growth of secondary tumour on the intrathecal nerve roots is not unusual. It is a common pattern of metastatic spread in medulloblastomas, for example, and is seen in meningiomatosis (Minckler, 1971). In patients with widespread carcinoma clinical symptoms of peripheral nerve damage are almost always the result of direct involvement of the nerve by tumour. 'Non-metastatic carcinomatous neuropathy' is seen in no more than 5 per cent of cases with malignant tumour and neuropathy (Harkin and Reed, 1959; see Chapter 5). An associated neuropathy is not unusual in Hodgkin's lymphogranulomatosis and in lymphosarcomas.

REFERENCES

Adair, F. E. and McLean, J. (1937). 'Tumors of the peripheral nerve system. With a report of 2782 cases.' In *Tumors of the Nervous System*, pp. 440–464. A.R.N.M.D.XVI. Baltimore; Williams and Wilkins.

D'Agostino, A. N., Soule, E. H. and Miller, R. H. (1963). 'Primary malignant neoplasms of nerves (malignant neurilemmomas) in patients without manifestations of multiple neurofibromatosis (von Recklinghausen's disease).' *Cancer,* **16,** 1003.

Antoni, N. (1920). *Über die Rückenmarkstumoren und Neurofibrome.* Munich; J. F. Bergmann.

Barber, K. W., Bianco, A. J., Soule, E. H. and MacCarty, C. S. (1962). 'Benign extraneural soft-tissue tumours of the extremities causing compression of nerves.' *J. Bone Joint Surg. A,* **44,** 98.

Barret, R. and Cramer, F. (1963). 'Tumors of the peripheral nerves and so-called "ganglia" of the peroneal nerve.' *Clin. Orthop.,* **27,** 135.

Beck, E. (1939). 'Zwei Fälle von Neurofibromatose mit Befallensein des ZNS.' *Z. Neurol. Psychiat.,* **164,** 748

Beckwith, J. B. and Martin, R. F. (1968). 'Observations on the histopathology of neuroblastoma.' *J. Pediat. Surg.,* **3,** 106.

Bernstein, J. J., Collins, G. H. and Bernstein, M. E. (1973). 'Ultrastructure of human spinal neuroma.' *J. Neurol. Sci.,* **18,** 489.

Bielschowsky, M. (1932). In *Cytology and Cellular Pathology of the Nervous System,* Vol. 3, p. 1083. Ed. by W. Penfield. New York: Paul B. Hoeber.

Bill, A. H. (1968). 'The regression of neuroblastoma.' *J. Pediat. Surg.,* **3,** 103.

Bolande, R. P. and Towler, W. F. (1970). 'A possible relationship of neuroblastoma to von Recklinghausen's disease.' *Cancer,* **26,** 162.

Braley, A. E. (1954). 'Medullated corneal nerves and plexiform neuroma associated with pheochromocytoma.' *Trans. Am. Ophthal. Soc.,* **52,** 189.

Carstens, H. B. and Schrodt, G. R. (1967). 'Malignant transformation of a benign encapsulated neurilemmoma.' *Am. J. Clin. Pathol.,* **51,** 144.

Cervós-Navarro, J. (1960). 'Elektronenmikroskopische Untersuchungen an Spinalganglienzellen. II. Satellitenzellen.' *Arch. Psychiat. Nervenk.,* **200,** 267.

Cervós-Navarro, J. (1969). 'Die Morphologie der hinteren Schädelgrube.' *Radiologe,* **9,** 458.

Cervós-Navarro, J., Bayer, J. M. and Käser, H. (1973). 'Ultrastrukturelle Differenzierung der Phäochromocytome.' *Virchows Arch. Abt. A, Pathol. Anat.,* **361,** 51.

Cervós-Navarro, J. and Matakas, F. (1975). 'The ultrastructure of reticulin.' *Acta Neuropath. (Berlin),* Suppl. IV, 173.

Cervós-Navarro, J., Matakas, F. and Lazaro, M. C. (1968). 'Das Bauprinzip der Neurinome. Ein Beitrag zur Histiogenese der Neurinome.' *Virchows Arch. Abt. A, Pathol. Anat.,* **345,** 276.

REFERENCES

Cervós-Navarro, J. and Stoltenbrug, G. (1976). 'Ultrastruktur mediastinaler und retroperitonealer Nerventumoren.' In preparation.

Cervós-Navarro, J. and Thies, W. (1976). In preparation.

Chapman, R. C., Kemp, V. E. and Taliaferro, I. (1959). 'Pheochromocytoma associated with multiple neurofibromatosis and intracranial hemangioma.' *Am. J. Med.,* **26,** 883.

Christensen, E. and Christensen, E. E. (1956). 'Medulloblastomas.' *Acta Psychiat. Neurol. Scand.,* **108,** 87.

Coriell, L. L. (1968). 'Host immunity.' *J. Pediat. Surg.,* **3,** 124.

Cravioto, R. (1969). 'The ultrastructure of acoustic nerve tumours.' *Acta Neuropath. (Berlin),* **12,** 116.

Cushing, H. and Wolbach, S. B. (1927). 'Transformation of malignant paravertebral sympathicoblastoma into benign ganglioneuroma.' *Am. J. Pathol.,* **3,** 203.

Dahl, E. V., Waugh, J. M. and Dahlin, D. C. (1957). 'Gastrointestinal ganglioneuromas. Brief review with a report of a duodenal ganglioneuroma.' *Am. J. Pathol.,* **33,** 953.

Daniell, H. W., Fazio, C. and Sacchi, U. (1954). 'Experimentally produced red softening of the brain.' *J. Neuropath. Exp. Neurol.,* **13,** 467.

Davis, F. W. Jr., Hull, J. G. and Vardell, J. C. Jr. (1950). 'Pheochromocytoma with neurofibromatosis.' *Am. J. Med.,* **8,** 131.

Döring, G. (1955). 'Pathologische Anatomie der Spinal-und Hirnnervenganglien, einschließlich der Wurzelnerven.' In *Handbuch der speziellen pathologischen Anatomie und Histologie,* Vol. 13, Part 5, pp. 249–356. Ed. by O. Lubarsch, F. Henke and R. Rössle.

van Epps, E. F., Hyndman, O. R. and Greene, J. A. (1964). 'Clinical manifestations of paroxysmal hypertension associated with pheochromocytoma of adrenal.' *Arch. Intern. Med.,* **65,** 1123.

Everson, T. C. and Cole, W. H. (1966). *Spontaneous Regression of Cancer.* Philadelphia; Saunders.

Feigin, I. (1971). 'The nerve sheath tumor, solitary and von Recklinghausen's disease; a unitary mesenchymal concept.' *Acta Neuropath. (Berlin),* **17,** 188.

Ferszt, R. (1975). 'Zur Morphologie des Rückenmarks im hohen Alter.' Dissertation, Berlin.

Fisher, E. R. and Wechsler, H. (1962). 'Granular cell myoblastoma—a misnomer. Electron microscopic and histochemical evidence concerning its Schwann cell derivation and nature (granular cell Schwannoma).' *Cancer,* **15,** 936.

Gardner, W. J. and Frazier, C. H. (1930). 'Bilateral acoustic neurofibromas: a clinical study and field survey of a family of five generations with a bilateral deafness in thirty-eight members.' *Arch. Neurol. (Chicago),* **23,** 266.

Gitlin, G. (1957). 'Concerning the gangliform enlargement (pseudoganglion on the nerve to the teres minor muscle).' *J. Anat.,* **91,** 466.

Gonzalez-Angulo, A., Reyes, H. A. and Navarrete Reyna, A. (1965). 'The ultrastructure of ganglioneuroblastoma. Observations on neoplastic ganglion cells.' *Neurology,* **15,** 242.

Gonzalez-Angulo, A., Smetana, K. and Martin, S. A. (1964). 'Estudio con microscopio electrónico de un caso de sarcoma neurógeno.' *Bol. Inst. Estud. Med. Biol. (Mex.),* **22,** 429.

Goldstein, M. (1966). 'Enzyme controlling the biosynthesis of catecholamines.' In *Neuroblastomas. Biochemical Studies,* p. 37. Ed. by C. Bohuon. Berlin; Springer.

Graham, W. D. and Johnston, C. R. (1957). 'Plantar digital neuroma.' *Lancet,* **273,** 470.

Greenfield, L. J. and Shelley, W. J. (1965). 'The spectrum of neurogenic tumors of the sympathetic nervous system: maturation and adrenergic function.' *J. Nat. Cancer Inst.,* **35,** 215.

Haller, F. R. and Low, F. N. (1971). 'The fine structure of the peripheral nerve root sheath in the subarachnoid space in the rat and other laboratory animals.' *Am. J. Anat.,* **131,** 1.

Harkin, J. C. and Reed, R. J. (1969). 'Tumors of the peripheral nervous system.' *Atlas of Tumor Pathology,* 2nd ser., Fasc. 3. Washington D.C.; Armed Forces Inst. Path.

Heard, G. (1962). 'Nerve sheath tumors in von Recklinghausen's disease of the nervous system.' *Ann. Roy. Coll. Surg. Engl.,* **31,** 229.

Hilding, D. A. and House, W. F. (1965). 'Acoustic neuroma: comparison of traumatic and neoplastic.' *J. Ultrastruct. Res.,* **12,** 611.

Hitchess, E. M. and Platt, D. S. (1972). 'Fibrosarcoma.' *Cancer,* **29,** 1369.

Hori, A. (1973). 'Intraspinale Schwannosen der Zona reticularis.' *Acta Neuropath. (Berlin),* **25,** 89.

Huber, C. G. and Lewis, D. (1920). 'Amputation neuromas.' *Arch. Surg.,* **1,** 85.

Isaacson, P. (1976). 'Mast cells in benign nerve sheath tumours.' *J. Pathol.,* **119,** 193.

Koop, C. E. (1968). 'Factors affecting survival in neuroblastoma.' *J. Pediat. Surg.,* **3,** 113.

REFERENCES

Krücke, W. (1974). 'Pathologie der peripheren Nerven.' In *Handbuch der Neurochirurgie*, Vol. 7, Part 3. Ed. by H. Olivecrona, W. Tönnis, and W. Krenkel. Berlin; Springer.

Lallemand, R. C. and Weller, R. O. (1973). 'Intraneural neurofibromas involving the posterior interosseous nerve.' *J. Neurol. Neurosurg. Psychiat.*, **36**, 991.

Losli, E. J. (1952). 'Intrinsic hemangiomas of peripheral nerves: report of two cases and review of literature.' *Arch. Pathol., (Berlin)*, **53**, 226.

Luse, S. (1960). 'Electron microscopic studies of brain tumors.' *Neurology*, **10**, 881.

Luse, S. A. (1964). 'Synaptic structures occurring in a neuroblastoma.' *Arch. Neurol. (Chicago)*, **11**, 185.

McCabe, J. S. and Low, F. N. 'The subarachnoid angle: an area of transition in peripheral nerve.' *Anat. Rec.*, **164**, 15.

Masson, P. (1942). 'Tumeurs encapsulées et bénignes des nerfs.' *Rev. Canad. Biol.*, **1**, 209.

Matakas, F. and Cervós-Navarro, J. (1969). 'Abwandlungen des Gewebsbildes der Neurinome im elektronenmikroskopischen Bild.' *Virchows Arch. Abt. A, Pathol. Anat.*, **347**, 160.

Matakas, F., Cervós-Navarro, J. Georgsson, G. and Waechter, R. V. (1971). 'Hiperplasia y neoplasia des las células de Schwann. Estudio ultraestructural.' *Arch. Fund. Roux-Ocefa*, **5**, 5.

Mathews, G. J. and Osterholm, J. L. (1972). 'Painful traumatic neuromas.' *Surg. Clinics N. Am.*, **51**, 1313.

Melicow, M. M. (1957). 'Hibernating fat and pheochromocytoma.' *Arch. Pathol. (Berlin)*, **63**, 367.

Minckler, J. (1971). 'Supporting cell tumors of peripheral nerves.' In *Pathology of the Nervous System*, Vol. II. Ed. by J. Minckler. New York; McGraw-Hill.

Misugi, K., Misugi, N. and Newton, W. A. Jr. (1968). 'Fine structural study of neuroblastoma, ganglioneuroblastoma, and pheochromocytoma.' *Arch. Pathol. (Berlin)*, **86**, 160.

Moscovic, E. A. and Azar, H. A. (1967). 'Multiple granular cell tumors ("myoblastomas").' *Cancer*, **20**, 2032.

Müller, W. (1965). 'Untersuchungen über die Lipoide im Neurinom.' *Verh. Dtsch. Ges. Pathol.*, **49**, 338.

Murray, Stout, A. P. (1942). 'Demonstration of the formation of reticulin by Schwannian cells *in vitro*.' *Am. J. Pathol.*, **18**, 585.

Naffziger, H. C. and Brown, H. A. (1933). 'Hour-glass tumours of the spine.' *Arch. Neurol. Psychiat.* **29**, 561.

Nathaniel, E. J. H. and Pease, D. C. (1963). 'Collagen and basement membrane formation by Schwann cells during nerve regeneration.' *J. Ultrastruct. Res.*, **9**, 550.

Nissen, K. I. (1951). 'The etiology of Morton's metatarsalgia.' *J. Bone Joint Surg.*, **33B**, 293.

Ochoa, J. and Neary, D. (1975). 'Localised hypertrophic neuropathy, intraneural tumour, or chronic nerve entrapment.' *Lancet*, March 15, 632.

Orcel, L., Luboinski, J. and Natali, J. (1972). 'Anatomic and histiogenetic study of rectal involvement in Recklinghausen's neurofibromatosis.' *Arch. Anat. Pathol. (Paris)*, **20**, 163.

Paquin, F. and Mandalenakis, N. (1973). 'Schwannome cellulaire dans le cadre d'une neurofibromatose. Etude histologique et ultrastructurale.' *Union Med. Can.*, **102**, 379.

Penfield, W. (1932). 'Tumours of the sheaths of the nervous system.' In *Cytology and Cellular Pathology of the Nervous System*, Vol. III, Sec. XIX, pp. 955–990. Ed. by W. Penfield. New York; Paul B. Hoeber.

Penfield, W. and Young, A. W. (1930). 'The nature of von Recklinghausen's disease and the tumors associated with it.' *Arch. Neurol. Psychiat. (Chicago)*, **23**, 320.

Perroncito, A. (1907). 'Die Regeneration der Nerven.' *Beitr. Pathol. Anat.*, **42**, 354.

Pick, L. and Bielschowsky, M. (1911). 'Über das System der Neurome und Beobachtungen an einem Ganglioneurom des Gehirns (nebst Untersuchungen über die Genese der Nervenfasern in Neurinomen).' *Z. Ges. Neurol. Psychiat.*, **6**, 391.

Pineda, A. (1965). 'Collagen formation by principal cells of acoustic tumours.' *Neurology*, **15**, 536.

Pineda, A. (1966). 'Electron microscopy of the tumor cells in "Neurofibromas".' *J. Neuropath. Exp. Neurol.*, **25**, 158.

Poirier, J. and Escourolle, R. (1967). 'Ultrastructure des neurinomes de l'acoustique.' *Z. Mikrosk.-Anat. Forsch.*, **76**, 509.

Poirier, J., Escourolle, R. and Castaigne, P. (1968). 'Les neurofibromes de la maladie de Recklinghausen.' *Acta Neuropath. (Berlin)*, **10**, 279.

Polak, M. (1950). 'Anatomia patológica y clasificación de los tumores de los nervios periféricos.' *Arch. Histol. (Buenos Aires)*, **4**, 103.

REFERENCES

Polak, M. (1966). 'Blastomas del sistema nervioso central y periférico.' In *Patologia y Ordenación Histogenética*. Buenos Aires; López Libreros Editores.

Preston, F. W., Walsh, W. S. and Clarke, T. H. (1952). 'Cutaneous neurofibromatosis (von Recklinghausen's disease): clinical manifestations and incidence of sarcoma in 61 male patients.' *Am. Med. Assoc. Arch. Surg.*, **64**, 813.

Rafel, S. S. G. (1962). 'Granular-cell myoblastoma.' *Oral Surg.*, **15**, 192.

Raimondi, A. J. and Beckmann, F. (1967). 'Perineurial fibroblastomas; their fine structure and biology.' *Acta Neuropath. (Berlin)*, **8**, 1.

Ramsey, H. J. (1965). 'Fibrous long-spacing collagen in tumours of the nervous system.' *J. Neuropath. Exp. Neurol.*, **24**, 40.

Rappaport, H. M. (1953). 'Neurofibromatosis of the oral cavity.' *Oral Surg.*, **6**, 599.

Raymond, F. (1893). 'Contribution à l'étude des Tumeurs neurologiques de la moelle epinière.' *Arch. Neurol. (Paris)*, **26**, 97.

Recklinghausen, von G. (1881). *Über die Beziehung der multiplen Fibrome der Haut zu den multiplen Neuromen*. Berlin; Hirschwald.

Riggs, H. E. and Clary, W. N. (1957). 'A case of intramedullary sheath cell tumor of the spinal cord.' *J. Neuropath. Exp. Neurol.*, **16**, 332.

Rio Hortega, P. del (1942). *Arch. Soc. Argent. Anat. Normal Patol.*, **1**, 4.

Rio Hortega, P. del (1942). *Arch. Soc. Argent. Anat. Normal Patol.*, **4**, 103.

Rio Hortega, P. del (1943). 'Carácteres e interpretación de las células especificas de los neurinomas (Schwannomas).' *Arch. Soc. Argent. Anat. Normal Patol.*, **5**, 103.

Robinson, R. (1966). 'Biochemical features of malignant tumors of sympathetic tissues.' In *Neuroblastomas. Biochemical Studies*, p. 66. Ed. by C. Bohuon. Berlin; Springer.

Röhlich, P. and Knopp, A. (1961). 'Electronenoptische Untersuchungen an den Hüllen des N. ischiadicus der Ratte.' *Z. Zellforsch.*, **53**, 299.

Rubinstein, L. J. (1963). 'Tumeurs et harmatomes dans la neurofibromatose centrale.' In L. Michaux and M. Feld, *Les Phakomatoses Cérébrales*. Paris; S.P.E.I.

Rubinstein, L. J. (1972). 'Tumors of the central nervous system.' *Atlas of Tumor Pathology*, 2nd Ser., Fasc. 6. Washington, D.C.; Armed Forces Inst. Pathol.

Russell, D. S. and Rubinstein, L. J. (1959). *Pathology of Tumours of the Nervous System*. London: Edward Arnold. Baltimore; Williams and Wilkins.

Russell, D. S. and Rubinstein, L. J. (1963). *Pathology of Tumours of the Nervous System*. London; Edward Arnold.

Sarin, C. L., Bennett, M. H. and Jackson, J. W. (1974). 'Intrathoracic neurofibroma of the vagus nerve.' *Br. J. Dis. Chest*, **68**, 46.

Scharenberg, K. (1971). 'Neurofibromatosis (von Recklinghausen's disease).' In *Pathology of the Nervous System* Vol. 2, pp. 1906–1916. Ed. by J. Minckler. New York; McGraw-Hill.

Schenkein, I., Bueker, E. D., Helson, L., Axelrod, F. and Dancis, J. (1974). 'Increased nerve-growth-stimulating activity in disseminated neurofibromatosis.' *New Engl. J. Med.*, March 14, 613.

Schmincke, A. (1956). 'Recklinghausensche Krankheit.' In *Handbuch der Spez. Path. Anatomie und Histologie*. Vol. 13, Part 4, pp. 664–695. Ed. by O. Lubarsch, F. Henke and R. Rössle. Berlin; Springer.

Schnitzler, L., Simard, C., Baudoux, D. and Lefranc, M. (1973). 'Cutaneous and mucosal neuromas, with a histopathologic and ultrastructural study.' *Ann. Dermatol. Syphilig. (Paris)*, **100**, 241.

Skydsgaard, H. (1944). 'Sympathoblastoma orbitae.' *Acta Neurol. Psychiat. Scand.*, **19**, 367.

Sobel, H. J., Marquet, E., Arvin, E. and Schwarz, R. (1971). 'Granular cell myoblastoma: An electron microscopic and cytochemical study illustrating the genesis of granules and ageing of myoblastoma cells.' *Am. J. Pathol.*, **65**, 59.

Staemmler, M. (1939). 'Beiträge zur normalen und pathologischen Anatomie des Rückenmarks.' *Z. Ges. Neurol. Psychiat.*, **164**, 669; *Z. Ges. Neurol. Psychiat.*, **166**, 529.

Stout, A. P. (1948). 'Fibrosarcoma. The malignant tumor of fibroblast.' *Cancer*, **1**, 30.

Stout, A. P. (1949). 'Tumors of the peripheral nervous system.' In *Atlas of Tumor Pathology*. Washington, D.C.; Armed Forces Inst. Pathol.

Stout, A. P. (1953). 'Tumors of the soft tissue.' In *Atlas of Tumor Pathology*, Sec. II, Fasc. 5. Washington, D.C.; Armed Forces Inst. Pathol.

Stowens, D. (1957). 'Neuroblastoma and related tumors.' *Arch. Pathol (Berlin)*, **63**, 451.

Tarlov, L. M. (1940). 'Origin of perineural fibroblastoma.' *Am. J. Pathol.*, **16**, 33.

Taylor, H. B. and Norris, H. J. (1967). 'Epithelial invasion of nerves in benign diseases of the breast.' *Cancer*, **20**, 2245.

206

REFERENCES

Tazawa, K., Soga, J. and Ito, H. (1970). 'Fine structure of neuroblastoma—a case report.' *Acta Pathol. Japon.*, **21** (2), 257.

Thies, W. (1964). 'Multiple echte fibrilläre Neurome (Rankenneurome) der Haut und Schleimhaut.' *Arch. Klin. Exp. Dermatol.*, **218**, 740.

Varon, S. (1968). 'Nerve growth factors in neuroblastoma pathology.' *J. Pediat. Surg.*, **3**, 120.

Verocay, J. (1908). *Multiple Geschwülste und Systemerkrankungen am nervösen Apparat.* Chiari Festschrift, Vienna and Leipzig.

Waggener, I. D. (1966). 'Ultrastructure of benign peripheral nerve sheath tumors.' *Cancer*, **19**, 699.

Webster, H. de F., Schröder, J. M., Asbury, A. K. and Adams, R. D. (1967). 'The role of the Schwann cells in the formation of "onion bulbs" found in chronic neuropathies.' *J. Neuropath. Exp. Neurol.*, **26**, 276.

Wechsler, W. and Hossmann, K. A. (1965). 'Zur Feinstruktur menschlicher Acusticusneurinome.' *Beitr. Pathol. Anat.*, **132**, 319.

Weller, R. O. (1974). '"Localised hypertrophic neuropathy" and hypertrophic polyneuropathy.' *Lancet*, **ii**, 592.

Williams, E. D. and Pollack, D. J. (1966). 'Multiple mucosal neuromata with endocrine tumours: a syndrome allied to von Recklinghausen's disease.' *J. Pathol. Bacteriol.*, **91**, 71.

Willis, R. A. (1959). *The Borderland of Embryology and Pathology.* London; Butterworths.

Willis, R. A. (1960). *Pathology of Tumors*, 4th edn. London; Butterworths.

Willis, R. A. (1972). *The Spread of Tumours in the Human Body.* London; Butterworths.

Yanagisawa, M. (1970). 'Electronmicroscopic study of neuroblastoma.' *Paediat. Univ. Tokyo*, **17**, 29.

Yokoyama, M., Okada, K., Takayasu, H. and Yamada, R. (1971). 'Ultrastructural and biochemical study of neuroblastoma and ganglioneuroblastoma.' *Invest. Urol.*, **9**, 156.

Yokoyama, M., Okada, K., Tokue, A. and Takayasu, H. (1973). 'Ultrastructural and biochemical study of benign ganglioneuroma.' *Virchows Arch. Abt. A, Pathol. Anat.*, **361**, 195.

Zülch, K. J. (1956). 'Biologie und Pathologie der Hirngeschwülste.' In *Handbuch der Neurochirurgie*, Vol. III. Ed. by H. Olivecrona and W. Tönnis. Berlin; Springer.

Zülch, K. J. (1963). 'Rapport entre les phakomatoses et la croissance initiale des tumeurs spontanées chez l'homme.' In *Les Phakomatoses Cérébrales*. Ed. by L. Michaux and M. Feld. Paris; S.P.E.I.

Appendix: A Guide to the Examination of Peripheral Nerve Biopsies

Before a peripheral nerve biopsy is examined it is important to be aware of the patient's full clinical picture and to have the results of biochemical, haematological and electrophysiological investigations. While the biopsy is being examined it is advisable to have a scheme for extracting the maximum amount of information from the biopsy.

Part 1 of this Appendix consists of a brief resumé, for the pathologist, of the major clinical signs and symptoms of peripheral nerve disease, and some of the investigations that may elucidate its pathology and aetiology. Part 2 is a guide to the general pathological features that are seen in peripheral nerve biopsies; this part also includes a number of special points that characterize certain neuropathies. Part 3 is a summary of the pathology in the major peripheral neuropathies.

PART 1. CLINICAL FEATURES IN PERIPHERAL NEUROPATHIES

Sensory neuropathies may be associated with pain, abnormal sensations and loss of sensory appreciation; often the extremities are more severely affected. Motor neuropathies are accompanied by muscle weakness and, in many cases, by muscle wasting. Autonomic involvement is characterized by postural hypotension, impotence, atonia of the bladder, etc.

The clinical history should reveal any family incidence of peripheral nerve disease as well as the age of onset and duration of the neuropathy. Examination of the patient will define the distribution of the neuropathy and establish whether only one nerve is affected (mononeuritis) or multiple nerves in an asymmetrical manner (mononeuritis multiplex), or whether there is the symmetrical distribution of a polyneuropathy. The sensory, motor or mixed sensorimotor character of the neuropathy should also be apparent.

Electromyography will often distinguish between primary muscle disease, on the one hand, and peripheral nerve and anterior horn cell disease, on the other. Nerve conduction velocities are usually only slightly reduced in neuropathies where there is mainly axonal degeneration, unless the damage to the nerve is extensive, when conduction may cease altogether. Gross slowing of nerve conduction is characteristic of segmental demyelinating neuropathies. Increased terminal latency is seen in electromyographic studies of 'dying back' neuropathies.

Examination of blood and CSF may provide useful information about the aetiology of peripheral nerve lesions, as may radiographic investigations.

PART 2. GENERAL PATHOLOGY OF PERIPHERAL NERVE LESIONS

This section is designed to assist in the extraction of the maximum amount of information from a nerve biopsy. In previous chapters the value of epoxy resin-embedding has been stressed, and in this section the major observations are based upon transverse sections of epoxy resin-embedded nerve stained with toluidine blue, with or without additional carbol fuchsin (left-hand column). Interpretation and possible further investigation is listed in the right-hand column. Details of histological techniques will be found in Chapter 2.

Observations in 1 μm epoxy resin transverse sections of nerve	Interpretation and further investigation
1. Is the nerve normal?	
(a) Normal numbers of large and small myelinated fibres.	*Check* teased fibres for normal internodal lengths. Sporadic short internodes suggest previous segmental demyelination. If all the internodes are short, this suggests previous axonal degeneration and regeneration.
(b) Non-myelinated fibres.	*Check* with electron microscope.
(c) Is the neuropathy mainly motor?	*Examine* muscle for denervation atrophy (see Chapter 2) and intramuscular nerves for 'dying back' neuropathy.
2. Is there any artefact?	
(a) Are the fascicles distorted?	
(b) Are the myelinated fibres distorted?	Interpret with caution.
3. Is there any evidence of axonal degeneration?	
(a) Oedema of the nerve, macrophages, myelin debris and loss of axons.	**Early axonal degeneration.** *Check* with teased fibres (fragmentation of axons and myelin). *Check* for Sudanophilic lipid in frozen sections.
(b) Axon balloons, clusters of thin, poorly myelinated axon sprouts.	**Regeneration.** *Check* with teased fibres: regenerated fibres have short internodes.
(c) Loss of small and large myelinated axons.	**Severe axonal degeneration with no regeneration.** *Check* with electron microscope for loss of non-myelinated fibres.
4. Is there selective loss of non-myelinated fibres?	**Amyloidosis.** *Check* for amyloid deposits. **Riley–Day syndrome** (familial dysautonomia). *Check* family history and assay nerve growth factor.

Observations in 1 μm *epoxy resin transverse sections of nerve*	*Interpretation and further investigation*
5. Is there segmental demyelination?	
(a) Oedema of nerve, macrophages, loss of myelin but preservation of axons.	**Early stages of segmental demyelination.** *Check* with teased fibres.
(b) Large axons with disproportionately thin myelin sheaths.	**Remyelination.** *Check* teased fibres for thin remyelinating internodes and for variation of internodal length along single fibres.
(c) Lymphocytic infiltration with segmental demyelination.	**Allergic segmental demyelination,** e.g. Guillain–Barré syndrome.
6. Are there 'onion-bulb' whorls?	
(a) Thinly myelinated, demyelinated, or normally myelinated axons surrounded by whorls of cellular processes.	**Hypertrophic neuropathy.** *Check* for segmental demyelination in teased fibres. *Check* for family history of neuropathy, or for personal history of recurrent or long-standing neuropathy.
7. Are there endoneurial deposits?	
(a) Amorphous Congo red positive blobs.	**Amyloidosis.** *Check* for gammopathy or family history.
(b) Abnormal lipid deposits in Schwann cells and macrophages; extensive segmental demyelination.	**Metachromatic leukodystrophy** (sulphatide lipidosis). *Check* for metachromatic lipid in frozen sections (cresyl violet and Hollander's stain). *Check* urine, blood and cultured fibroblasts for arylsulphatase A levels.
(c) Crystalline deposits in Schwann cells and foamy macrophages.	**Krabbe's globoid cell leukodystrophy** (? sulphotransferase deficiency).
(d) Single, whorl-like bodies composed of collagen and fibroblasts.	**Renaut bodies:** present in normal nerves.
8. Are there granulomata in the nerve?	**Sarcoid.** *Check* for sarcoid granulomata elsewhere. **Leprosy.** *Check* for **Mycobacterium leprae.**
9. Is the perineurium thickened?	Possibly previous trauma.
10. Are there lipid deposits in the perineurium?	
(a) Birefringent lipid with lamellated ultrastructure.	**Fabry's disease.** *Check* skin lesions for confirmation of diagnosis.
11. Are the vessels abnormal?	Small neural vessels may be normal when the ischaemic neuropathy is due to atherosclerosis of larger arteries.
(a) Active vasculitis: lymphocytic cuffing, medial necrosis, thrombotic occlusion.	**Polyarteritis nodosa** and other collagen diseases. *Check* appearances in paraffin sections and elastic stain. *Check* for immune complexes in the vessel wall.

Observations in 1 μm epoxy resin transverse sections of nerve	Interpretation and further investigation
(b) Proliferative endarteritis; revascularized lumen.	**Old arteritic lesions** of polyarteritis, rheumatoid neuropathy, etc.
(c) Infiltration of vessel wall by Congo red positive material	**Amyloidosis.** *Check* type of amyloidosis.

PART 3. SUMMARY OF PATHOLOGICAL FEATURES IN THE MAJOR GROUPS OF PERIPHERAL NEUROPATHIES

A. Spinal cord disorders, motor neurone disease and spinal muscular atrophies

Mainly the motor nerve fibres are affected (axonal degeneration) unless the dorsal roots or ganglia are also involved. *Check* for denervation atrophy in muscle biopsies.

B. Peroneal muscular atrophy and hypertrophic neuropathy

A group of mainly hereditary diseases with loss of motor fibres, denervation atrophy of distal limb muscles and collateral sprouting of intramuscular nerves. Several types have segmental demyelination and hypertrophic neuropathy involving sensory nerves.

C. Friedreich's ataxia

Commonest form of hereditary ataxia. Loss of large myelinated fibres from sensory nerves (axonal degeneration).

D. Hereditary sensory neuropathies

Axonal degeneration in sensory nerves due to loss of neurones in sensory ganglia. There is a deficiency of non-myelinated fibres in familial dysautonomia. There may be widespread autonomic dysfunction.

E. Peripheral neuropathies in disorders of lipid metabolism

(i) There is segmental demyelination and accumulation of sulphatide in Schwann cells and endoneurial macrophages in **metachromatic leukodystrophy**; diagnosis is confirmed by reduced arylsulphatase A levels in urine, blood and cultured fibroblasts metachromatic granules in urine.

211

(ii) Segmental demyelination is seen in **Krabbe's globoid leukodystrophy** (cerebroside sulphotransferase deficiency); crystalline Schwann cell deposits and foamy macrophages are seen in the nerves.

(iii) Loss of myelinated fibres (axonal degeneration) and glycolipid deposits in the perineurium are seen in **Fabry's disease** (angiokeratoma corporis diffusum) due to deficiency of ceramide trihexosidase. Diagnosis is confirmed by biopsy of skin lesions.

(iv) Hypertrophic neuropathy is seen in **Refsum's disease** where there is a deficiency in metabolism of the fatty acid, phytanic acid; high levels of phytanic acid are found in the serum.

F. Amyloidosis

Peripheral neuropathy occurs in familial amyloidosis, primary amyloidosis and amyloidosis associated with B-lymphocyte dyscrasias, but rarely in secondary amyloidosis. The carpal tunnel syndrome is associated with amyloid deposition in the flexor retinaculum. Amyloid in the endoneurium and in vessel walls is seen in other types of amyloidosis and results in axonal degeneration, often with selective loss of non-myelinated fibres.

G. Neuropathy in acute intermittent porphyria

A 'dying back' neuropathy affecting predominantly distal ends of the large motor fibres in proximal muscles.

H. Trauma and compression

Mild degrees of trauma or compression may cause segmental demyelination only. More severe trauma leads to axonal degeneration distal to the site of injury. Biopsy of the affected nerve may reveal early or late stages of axonal degeneration, or axonal regeneration (see Part 2), depending upon the timing of the biopsy.

I. Neuropathies due to vascular disease

Mild ischaemia often results in primary segmental demyelination; axonal degeneration and even local infarction of the nerve are seen in severe vascular disease. Atheroma of the limb arteries may be accompanied by axonal degeneration in the limb nerves.

Vasculitis and thrombotic occlusion of the vasa nervorum occurs in a variety of collagen and immune complex diseases. Patchy axonal degeneration is seen in the peripheral nerves; thus, the axonal loss is usually most severe in the distal parts of the nerve.

J. Toxic neuropathies

Toxic substances mostly cause 'dying back' neuropathies with degeneration of the distal portions of the long, large-diameter motor nerve fibres. Segmental demyelination occurs in some toxic neuropathies, e.g. those due to lead and diphtheria toxin. Other substances, e.g. botulinum and tetanus toxins, affect the motor nerve terminals.

K. Metabolic neuropathies

(i) *Diabetes.* Numerically a very important neuropathy which often involves sensory nerves. Segmental demyelination and sometimes 'onion-bulb' formation (hypertrophic neuropathy) are seen. Axonal degeneration occurs in more chronic cases.

(ii) *Vitamin deficiencies.* Mainly 'dying-back' neuropathies.

(iii) *Uraemic neuropathies.* Axonal degeneration in the distal sensory nerves.

L. Inflammatory diseases

(i) *Acute post-infections polyneuritis (Guillain–Barré syndrome).* Allergic segmental demyelination with widespread infiltration of affected nerve fascicles by macrophages, lymphocytes and plasma cells. Remyelination is seen during the recovery stage, and 'onion-bulb' formation may be present in recurrent cases. Axonal degeneration occurs in severe cases.

(ii) *Virus infections.* Axonal degeneration and denervation atrophy are seen in the affected nerves and muscles in poliomyelitis due to loss of anterior horn cells. Varicella zoster virus may be seen by electron microscopy or immunofluorescence in the skin lesions and sensory ganglia together with accumulation of mononuclear cells. Fibrosis of the ganglion and axonal degeneration of the nerve may be seen in herpes zoster.

(iii) *Leprosy.* Numerous *Mycobacterium leprae* are seen in Schwann cells and some in axons in **lepromatous leprosy**; this is accompanied by axonal degeneration and fibrosis of the nerves.

Nodular thickening and destruction of the architecture of the nerve by granulomata is characteristically seen in **tuberculoid leprosy**. There is extensive axonal degeneration especially in the cutaneous nerves. Few *M. leprae* are present. Intermediate forms of leprosy are common.

(iv) *Sarcoidosis.* Sarcoid granulomata are occasionally seen in nerve.

M. Neuropathy in malignant disease

Nerves may be damaged by direct spread of primary or metastatic tumour resulting in segmental demyelination and axonal degeneration.

Non-metastatic effects include myopathy and encephalopathy. Peripheral neuropathies vary in their severity; they show a mixture of segmental demyelination and axonal degeneration. Lymphocytic infiltration of the affected nerves may be seen.

N. Neuropathies in the aged

The cumulative effect of axonal degeneration and segmental demyelination from 'wear and tear' throughout life may contribute to the high incidence of peripheral nerve signs in the aged. In addition, other diseases, e.g. vascular and malignant disease, may affect older people.

O. Autonomic neuropathies

Autonomic neuropathies occur as part of several neuropathies, e.g. diabetes, amyloid, Fabry's disease and familial dysautonamia, and occasionally as distinct syndromes. In some, degeneration of neurones in the autonomic nervous system has been described.

P. Myasthenia gravis

The main pathological findings are bizarre and disordered arborizations of the intramuscular nerve terminals and simplification of the muscle end-plate ultrastructure. Lymphocytic infiltration of muscle and neurogenic atrophy may also be seen.

THE BRITISH SCHOOL OF OSTEOPATHY
1-4 SUFFOLK STREET, LONDON SW1Y 4HG
TEL: 01-930 9254-8

Index